Infection Control
in Respiratory Care

Second Edition

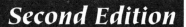

Arthur J. McLaughlin, Jr., MS, CRTT
Former Director of Respiratory Care
Wilmington Medical Center
Wilmington, Delaware
President
A.J. McLaughlin and Associates
Wilmington, Delaware

with
Roberto Palermo, BA, MBA, RRT, CPFT
Manager, Respiratory Care Department
Union Hospital
Elkton, Maryland

Illustrations by
Louis Bieda

20977

An Aspen Publication®
Aspen Publishers, Inc.
Gaithersburg, Maryland
1996

Library of Congress Cataloging-in-Publication Data

McLaughlin, Arthur J., 1947–
Infection control in respiratory care / by Arthur J. McLaughlin ;
with Roberto Palermo ; illustrations by Louis Bieda. — 2nd ed.
p.   cm.
Rev. ed. of: Manual of infection control in respiratory care. 1st
ed. c1983.
Includes bibliographical references and index.
ISBN 0-8342-0787-7
1. Respiratory infections—Prevention.   2. Nosocomial infections-
-Prevention.   3. Respiratory therapy.   I. Palermo, Roberto.
II. McLaughlin, Arthur J., 1947–   Manual of infection control in
respiratory care. III. Title.
[DNLM: 1. Cross Infection—prevention & control.   2. Respiratory
Care Units—standards.   3. Sterilization—methods.   4. Respiratory
Tract Diseases.   WX 167 M478i 1996]
RC740.M35   1996
616.2—dc20
DNLM/DLC
for Library of Congress
96-21362
CIP

Aspen Publishers, Inc., grants permission for photocopying for limited personal or internal use.
This consent does not extent to other kinds of copying, such as copying for general distribution, for
advertising or promotional purposes, for creating new collective works, or for resale. For
information, address Aspen Publishers, Inc., Permissions Department, 200 Orchard Ridge Drive,
Suite 200, Gaithersburg, Maryland 20878.

Orders: (800) 638-8437
Customer Service: (800) 234-1660

About Aspen Publishers • For more than 35 years, Aspen has been a leading professional publisher in a variety of disciplines. Aspen's vast information resources are available in both print
and electronic formats. We are committed to providing the highest quality information available
in the most appropriate format for our customers. Visit Aspen's Internet site for more information
resources, directories, articles, and a searchable version of Aspen's full catalog, including the
most recent publications: http://www.aspenpub.com
Aspen Publishers, Inc. • The hallmark of quality in publishing
Member of the worldwide Wolters Kluwer group

The authors have made every effort to ensure the accuracy of the information herein. However,
appropriate information sources should be consulted, especially for new or unfamiliar
procedures. It is the responsibility of every practitioner to evaluate the appropriateness of a
particular opinion in the context of actual clinical situations and with due considerations to new
developments. Authors, editors, and the publisher cannot be held responsible for any
typographical or other errors found in this book.

Editorial Resources: Greg Balas
Library of Congress Catalog Card Number: 96-21362
ISBN: 0-8342-0787-7

Printed in the United States of America

1   2   3   4   5

Dedicated to
Bill Scott, RRT
for years of unswerving support and friendship

What, will these hands ne'er be clean?

William Shakespeare, *Macbeth*

Table of Contents

Preface

The first edition of *Manual of Infection Control in Respiratory Care* was written in 1983 to provide respiratory-care practitioners with a convenient and concise reference regarding aseptic procedures and emphasizing the careful processing of respiratory-care equipment. A short review of microbiology was included and the importance of hand washing was stressed.

The second edition presents the subject of infection control in respiratory care in a manner that reflects the dramatic changes in both the complexity and importance of aseptic practices that have evolved since 1983. The information herein is based on the rationale behind the development of universal blood and body fluid precautions and new knowledge in the field of infectious diseases from an environmental systems point of view.

A new chapter, "Concepts in Infectious Disease," presents basic concepts in the understanding of the transmission of diseases and epidemiology in the community. These concepts are then integrated into an expanded and updated discussion of hospital infections in the next chapter, "Nosocomial Infections."

The chapter, "Review of Microbiology," now comprises nearly half of the book in response to the fact that respiratory-care practitioners treat patients who have a great variety of infectious diseases, including opportunistic infections, superinfections, and antimicrobial-resistant infections. Therefore, it covers many more bacterial and viral organisms than were addressed in the first edition. Also, discussions of fungal diseases and animal parasites have been added as well as tables that list important antimicrobial agents. Characteristics of diseases that are caused by specific microorganisms are described. These characteristics include symptoms, treatment, prevention, and epidemiology of diseases and follow the model developed by Robert F. Boyd, PhD and Bryan Hoerl, PhD Diseases of special importance or interest to respiratory-care practitioners, as well as possible cardiopulmonary complications that result from all the discussed diseases are stressed. Thus, the chapter has been renamed, "Review of Medical Microbiology." In keeping with these changes, the glossary has been revised and enlarged.

The chapter, "Aseptic Techniques," in this edition, begins with a short history of the attempts to control nosocomial infections in the United States and goes on to explain the development of current isolation and universal blood and body fluids precautions. Emphasis on the rationale behind specific isolation precautions and specific universal precautions is included in the presentation of mandated, or recommended, policies. The hospital is presented as a special environment in which many respiratory-therapy practitioners function.

Throughout, the text reflects changes in the techniques and modalities of therapy that are used in respiratory care, keeping in mind that modalities vary with types of institutions and geographical locations; thus discussions of equipment present general principles that are intended to apply to categories of equipment. Suggestions for the design of processing areas for respiratory-care equipment have been updated as a result of changes and to be in accordance with current standards and recommendations for aeration and ventilation. Recommendations for the level of asepsis necessary for specific items used in respiratory care follow both E.H. Spaulding's classification system and the guidelines from the Centers for Disease Control and Prevention.

Finally, for this edition, the word *manual* has been dropped from the title for two reasons. The first reason is in recognition of the fact that individual institutions and departments develop procedures and manuals tailored to their own needs and patient populations that follow the guidelines of the Centers for Disease Control and the mandates from the Occupational Health and Safety Administration as well as the recommendations of many professional groups. The second reason is because the developments in the field of infectious disease control worldwide have caused both the scope and approach of this book to be changed in order to provide respiratory-care practitioners and students with more information about infectious diseases as well as a broader overview of the role of microorganisms in both the general environment and the hospital environment. While some of the information in this book will be well known to experienced practitioners, it was written with the needs of students and beginning practitioners in mind.

In this edition, hand washing is once again stressed many times because its importance in preventing the spread of disease cannot be overstated.

Acknowledgments

I would never have undertaken to write a book on this subject had I not had the opportunity to learn from the eminent Elvyn Scott, MS, MT (ASCP), who patiently instructed me for years.

I thank my editor, Steve Zollo and Aspen Publishers, Inc., for this opportunity and Mary Anne Langdon for walking me through the process. I also thank Bob Lang, RRT; Mary Lang, MS, RN; Joe Ciarlo, RRT; Tom Blackson, RRT; and Dave Ayars, CRTT, for advice and support. I thank Dave Spilver for 20 years as my editor, agent, and friend. Final thanks go to my brother Greg, and to my mother for proofreading the manuscript and to Suzie and Lizzie for helping me in all ways.

Chapter 1

Concepts in Infectious Disease

CHAPTER OBJECTIVES

Upon completion of this chapter, the reader will be able to

1. differentiate between the concepts of colonization and infection
2. describe the four stages of acute disease
3. differentiate between direct and indirect transmission of disease
4. contrast and compare horizontal and vertical transmission of disease

I. Basic Concepts

A host is the organism from which a parasite derives its nourishment, and microscopic parasites may be intracellular or extracellular. Colonization implies the presence of a microorganism in or on the host with growth and multiplication of the microorganism but without any overt symptoms or detected immune reaction at the time it is isolated. An infection is the process wherein the host, after contact with microorganisms, responds by producing antibodies. *Disease* refers to tissue damage that is caused by the microorganism after infection takes place. Microorganisms that are able to cause disease are referred to as pathogenic. Virulence is a measure of the organism's disease-producing potential and is related to the organism's ability to invade tissue or to produce toxins. Loss of virulence in an organism is referred to as attenuation. People who harbor pathogenic organisms but do not have symptoms of disease are referred to as carriers. Both pathogenicity and virulence vary as a result of two groups of factors: host factors and microbial factors.

1

A. Host Factors
   1. The body site that affords entry of microorganisms is referred to as the portal of entry and includes the skin, mucosal surfaces, respiratory tract, oropharynx, intestinal tract, and genitourinary tract.
   2. Other host factors include the immunological status, genetic constitution, age, race, sex, nutritional status, occupation, and underlying health conditions.
B. Microbial Factors
   Microbial factors include the ability of the microorganism to adhere to host tissue, to penetrate the epithelium, and to produce exotoxins and/or endotoxins. Microbial factors also include the microorganism's antiphagocytic ability, antigenic variability, and serum resistance. The type of organism involved, the infectious dose, or the number of organisms involved in the infection are additional microbial factors.

II. Stages of Disease

When an infection can be inhibited by a host's immune system to the extent that symptoms are negligible or absent, it is referred to as being subclinical or inapparent. If an infection develops to the disease state, it is termed either acute or chronic.

A. Acute disease produces symptoms that usually appear quickly, become intense, and then subside. The disease process can further be divided into periods that are more easily identified in acute disease.
   1. The incubation period is the time between entry of the infectious agent and the appearance of symptoms. This period may range from a few hours to several years.
   2. The prodromal period refers to the symptoms experienced rather than the actual time involved. The symptoms are those of malaise, which can include headache, upset stomach, low fever, and a sense of not feeling well.
   3. The acute period refers to the time that symptoms are at their peak.
   4. The convalescent period refers to the recovery phase, in which symptoms decline sharply.
B. Chronic disease produces symptoms that are experienced over a long time and may occur in periods of relapse.

III. Reservoirs and Sources of Disease

Reservoirs of infectious agents are places, animate or inanimate, where microorganisms live and multiply. Sources of infectious agents are objects or places, animate or inanimate, from which infection occurs. A reservoir and source in a given situation may be the same.

A. Animate Reservoirs
    1. The most important animate reservoir is the human body. Many viruses and bacteria utilize the human body as their only reservoir. Carriers (human reservoirs) may be either convalescent carriers, those who are recovering from a disease without symptoms, or healthy carriers, those who do not have disease but are carrying infectious organisms.
    2. Animals are important reservoirs and sources of disease for human beings. Domestic animals, such as poultry, cattle, and swine play particularly important roles in human infection. Diseases that normally occur in animals but that can be transmitted to human beings are called zoonoses.
    3. Insects, particularly arthropods, that transfer infectious microorganisms from one host to another are referred to as vectors. Mechanical vectors carry infectious agents on their bodies, while biological vectors serve as hosts for infectious agents themselves and infect other hosts while feeding on their blood.
B. Inanimate Reservoirs
    1. Many microorganisms, especially fungi, carry out their life cycles in soil. Human infection can result from contact with soil containing fungi (especially spores) and bacterial species that are indigenous to the soil.
    2. Water contains organic matter that supports microbial life. In addition, water is often contaminated by sewage containing pathogens.
    3. Food is an important reservoir for pathogenic microorganisms. Meat, milk, eggs, and other foods can be infected as they are produced, processed, or handled as they are prepared for cooking. Shellfish can also be contaminated by the water in which they grow.

IV. Disease Transmission

Infectious microorganisms are transferred from sources to hosts in three basic ways:

A. Contact

1. Direct contact refers to the transmission of microorganisms from person to person, usually via handshaking, kissing, sneezing, coughing, and sexual contact. Direct contact also includes the situation wherein a person transfers his own indigenous species from one body site to another, resulting in infection, and is referred to as an endogenous infection.

2. Indirect transmission refers to person-to-person transmission via an intermediate object, such as food, water, or dust. Objects that transfer microorganisms other than food and water are called fomites and can be almost any physical object.

   a. Water can transfer microorganisms through drinking, contact with abraded skin, inhalation or aspiration, and contact with mucous membranes.

   b. Food can transfer microorganisms if it is obtained in the contaminated state, is not kept at proper temperatures, is contaminated by food preparers, contacts contaminated equipment, e.g., meat grinders, or is inadequately cooked.

      (1) Food infection results from ingesting microorganisms.

      (2) Food poisoning results from ingesting toxins produced by microorganisms.

   c. Fomites are frequently implicated in the spread of disease in the community and in hospitals.

B. Air

Although air does not act as a reservoir, microorganisms are spread through the air on wind currents for distances farther than those involved in sneezing and coughing. Indoors, microorganisms are spread (disseminated) in dust or droplet nuclei (particles of mucus 5 μm or smaller) or in aerosols generated by humidifying devices or cooling towers.

C. Vectors

Vectors are important in community-related infections, though they are rarely involved in hospital-related infections (see III, A, 3).

V. Horizontal and Vertical Transmission

Microorganisms are spread from one person to another in one of two general fashions.

A. Horizontal transmission occurs when disease is transmitted through everyday contact, i.e., direct contact, vectors, air, water, or fomites.

B. Vertical transmission occurs when disease is transmitted from parent to offspring via sperm, ovum, placenta, milk, or direct contact. Transmission may occur postnatally, congenitally, or perinatally.

VI. Disease in the Community

Infectious diseases are seen in a given community or population at different frequencies, depending on many factors.

A. Endemic disease refers to a situation wherein a given disease exists in a specified population at a relatively constant rate.

B. Increased numbers of cases of disease above a normal endemic level are referred to as epidemic. The term *pandemic* refers to worldwide epidemics.

C. Sporadic diseases are those that occur in irregular patterns. The term *incidence* (of disease) refers to the number of new cases in a given population within a given time. This number is also referred to as the morbidity rate, while the number of deaths caused by the disease is called the mortality rate.

D. The total number of cases, both new and old, in the population within a given time is called the *prevalence* of the disease.

E. The term *herd immunity* refers to the situation in which a number of individuals in a given population are immune to a disease, whether acquired naturally or artificially, and thus prevent the rapid spread of the disease in that population. This is an important concept in the practice of immunization for specific diseases.

F. The surveillance of disease in a community, done in order to show its distribution, is called descriptive epidemiology. Four facts about an outbreak of disease are usually recorded. The first fact to be recorded is the host factors (see I, A). The second fact is the place, or physical location of the outbreak. The third fact usually recorded is time, or the season in which the outbreak takes place. Finally, the fourth fact that is recorded is the number of reported cases that is then plotted against time to develop a curve called an epidemic curve. The curve begins with the first reported case, the index case, and produces one of two classical curves. Common-source epidemics exhibit a sharp rise in cases with a gradual tapering off in cases, while contact-spread epidemics exhibit a slower rise and a flatter peak.

SUGGESTED READING

Baron, S., ed. *Medical Microbiology,* 3d ed. New York: Churchill Livingstone, 1991.

Boyd, R. F. *Basic Medical Microbiology,* 5th ed. Boston: Little Brown, 1995.

Hoeprich, P. D., M. C. Jordan, and A. R. Ronald. *Infectious Diseases,* 5th ed. Philadelphia: J. B. Lippincott, 1994.

Howard, B. J. *Clinical and Pathogenic Microbiology,* 2d ed. St. Louis: Mosby-Yearbook, 1994.

Chapter 2

Nosocomial Infections

CHAPTER OBJECTIVES

Upon completion of this chapter, the reader will be able to

1. discuss the impact of nosocomial infections on health care in the United States
2. explain why some nosocomial infections are classified as nonpreventable
3. contrast the concepts of epidemic and outbreak
4. describe three major links in the "chain of infection"
5. discuss the importance of gram-negative bacteria in nosocomial infections
6. discuss at least three factors that make the hospital a special environment relative to the spread of infections
7. discuss the functions of an employee health service

Nosocomial infections are infections that develop within a hospital or are produced by microorganisms acquired during hospitalization. They are a major threat to the health of hospitalized patients. The inability to reduce effectively the rate of patients' nosocomial infections increases the length of their hospital stay and results in substantially higher health care costs, estimated to be more than $4 billion per year. It is estimated that 2 million nosocomial infections occur in the United States each year.

It is believed that these infections cause more than 20 000 deaths directly and contribute to 60 000 more deaths. If all of these deaths were counted as part of mortality statistics, nosocomial infections would rate

7

as the fourth leading cause of death behind heart disease, cancer, and stroke. It is the responsibility of all health care workers to reduce the incidence of nosocomial infection through the use of proper aseptic techniques (those designed to avoid infection).

The term *nosocomial* (from the Greek, *noso,* meaning disease; and *komeion,* meaning care for) *infection* applies not only to infections that develop in patients, but also to infections that develop in anyone as a result of having had contact with a hospital. This includes visitors, health care workers, hospital maintenance workers, dietary staff, housekeeping staff, volunteers, salespersons, and so forth.

I. Nosocomial Symptoms

Most nosocomial infections in patients produce symptoms while the patients are hospitalized, but some do not.

A. As many as 25% of postoperative wound infections become symptomatic after the patients have been discharged. This occurs when patients are colonized or infected while in the hospital, but the incubation period is longer than the patient's hospital stay. Hepatitis B is an example of a disease that produces no symptoms until long after the patient is discharged.

B. Infections that are incubating at the time that a patient is admitted to a hospital are not classified as nosocomial but rather as community acquired, unless they were acquired during a previous admission.

C. Nosocomial infections are classified as being one of two types: preventable and nonpreventable.

1. Preventable infections are those that could have been prevented if some event related to the infection had been altered. The classic and most frequent example of this type of infection is when health care workers do not wash their hands after contact with a patient. Thirty percent of nosocomial infections are classified as preventable.

2. Nonpreventable infections are those that occur despite all possible precautions. An example is the situation in which immunosuppressed patients are infected by their own flora.

D. Hospital epidemics, especially common-vehicle (multiple infections caused by contact with a contaminated object) infections, are potentially preventable, but epidemics account for only a small percentage of the total number of nosocomial infections. Endemic infections produce the majority of nosocomial infections.

II. The Sources of Nosocomial Infections

A. Endogenous infections are caused by patients' own flora. The microorganisms involved may have been brought into the hospital with the patient or may have been acquired during the hospital stay. Endogenous infections are often the result of surgical manipulation, chemotherapy, and diagnostic or therapeutic procedures, and in those cases are referred to as *iatrogenic* infections.

B. Exogenous infections result from the transmission of organisms from a source other than the patient.

C. If it is not possible to determine if an infection is caused by an organism that is endogenous or exogenous, the term *autogenous* is used.

III. Hospital Epidemiology

The key to determining if a nosocomial infection problem exists in a particular situation is to track the frequency of cases that are currently reported and contrast that to the history of disease in the institution. Frequency is characterized as

- sporadic, or occurring occasionally and irregularly, with no specific pattern
- endemic, or occurring with ongoing frequency in a specific area, in a specific population, and over a specified time
- hyperendemic, or gradually increasing in a specific area beyond the expected number of cases
- epidemic, or showing a definite increase beyond endemic levels

A. *Outbreak* is a term sometimes used interchangeably with *epidemic,* but is also used to indicate an increased rate of occurrence, not yet at the epidemic level.

B. The occurrence of infection is defined by two concepts: incidence and prevalence (see Chap. 1, VI, C and D)

C. The three techniques used in epidemiologic studies are descriptive epidemiology (see Chap. 1, VI, F); analytic epidemiology, which is the study of disease distribution in terms of possible causal relationships; and experimental epidemiology, which is a method of proving or disproving a hypothesis about an outbreak.

IV. The Chain of Infection

An essential concept in the control of nosocomial infection is that of the chain of infection, which states that there are three factors, agent, transmission, and host, in the infection process. These factors are interrelated, and their relationship lies at the root of the transmission of disease from the infectious agent to the host. This relationship is called the ecology of infection, and attempts at controlling the ecology are based on attacking the weakest link of the chain.

A. The infectious agent, the first link in the chain of infection, may be a bacterium, virus, fungus, or parasite. Factors related to the host include pathogenicity, reservoirs and sources, and a period of infectivity.

1. Pathogenicity

   a. Pathogenicity is the measure of the ability of a microorganism to produce disease (see Chap. 1, I).

   b. Virulence, which is a measure of the severity of the disease, is based on the morbidity, mortality, and communicability of the disease. This measure ranges from slight to high.

   c. Invasiveness relates to the ability of a microorganism to invade tissues.

   d. The infectious dose (ID50) refers to the number of organisms necessary to produce disease, which varies from organism to organism and is influenced by the mode of transmission.

   e. Specificity refers to the number of hosts in which the microorganism can exist, e.g., human beings and cattle, or rats, mice, and human beings.

2. Reservoirs and sources (see Chap. 1, III)

   a. A reservoir is a place where an organism metabolizes and replicates. Viruses survive better in human reservoirs than do gram-positive bacteria, but gram-negative bacteria may have human, animal, or inanimate reservoirs.

   b. Sources are places from which an infectious agent passes to a host by direct, or indirect, contact, or through a vehicle. Sources may also be animate or inanimate. A source may be mobile or fixed; that is, patients may be trans-

ported to the source, e.g., a whirlpool bath, or the source may be transported to the patient, e.g., medical equipment.
3. Period of infectivity
The manner in which organisms exit the human body is important in the transmission of disease. The major portals of exit are the respiratory and gastrointestinal tracts, skin, wounds, and blood.

B. Transmission is the second link in the chain of infection and refers to the movement of organisms from source to host, which may occur via one or more of four routes.
1. Contact spread (see Chap. 1, IV, A, B, and C)
a. Direct-contact spread refers to person-to-person spread through physical contact, e.g., by touching. The most effective method of reducing the incidence of contact spread of infections in the hospital is strict adherence to hand washing procedures.
b. Indirect contact spread involves a physical object's being passively involved in the transmission of disease, e.g., a bronchoscope.
c. Droplet spread refers to the spread of organisms a short distance (several feet) through the air where they can contact people directly, or they can settle on surfaces where they remain infectious. Droplet spread is the result of sneezing, talking, or coughing. Streptococcal pharyngitis is a droplet-spread infection.
2. Common-vehicle spread
This type of infection occurs when a contaminated inanimate vehicle is responsible for the infection of multiple persons, e.g., food, blood, and blood products. Many vehicles can be contaminated from a common source, each time producing multiple infections. Conversely, a common source can contaminate many vehicles.
3. Airborne spread
This type of infection occurs when organisms are airborne for a distance of several feet and involves droplet nuclei (5 μm or smaller), dust particles, or skin squames. The classic example of airborne spread by droplet nuclei is the dissemination of tuberculosis. Airborne spread through skin squames occurs when healthy human beings every day lose a substantial number of desquamated epithelial cells that often carry *S.*

aureus organisms. Another airborne spread involves individuals with eczema who lose even more cells with potentially more infectious organisms on them.

4. Vector-borne spread (see Chap. 1, III, A, 3)

The spread of nosocomial disease involving vectors is thought not to occur in the United States, but such spread is theoretically possible.

C. The host is the third factor in the chain of infection (see Chap. 1, I, A)

1. Entrance (portal of entry)

The site of a microorganism's entry into a host is important in the progress of any infection. An organism may colonize one site, for example, and not cause disease, but at another site, disease results, e.g., *E. coli* in the intestinal tract may not cause disease, but in the urinary tract may cause disease.

2. Nonspecific defense mechanisms

The nonspecific defense mechanisms include the skin, mucous membranes and mucous, tears, gastrointestinal acid, enzymes, peristalsis, cilia, and local inflammatory responses.

3. Specific defense mechanisms

The specific defense mechanisms include natural immunity, artificial immunity (either actively, through vaccination, or passively, through serum globulin), acquired immunity, and transplacental antibody immunity.

4. Environmental factors

The environment can play a role in the ability of organisms to reproduce or be spread through the air and can also affect a host's resistance, e.g., excessively dry air can cause mucous membranes to dry and become susceptible to infection.

D. Factors that predispose patients to infection vary.

1. Age as a factor

a. Very young children, especially premature babies, are extremely susceptible to infection, especially *E. coli,* which causes neonatal sepsis. Children are highly susceptible until the age of six to *Haemophilus influenzae.*

b. Older patients with existing cardiovascular disease, respiratory disease, or urinary-tract abnormalities are very prone to contracting nosocomial infections.

2. Metabolic disorders as factors
   a. Patients with leukemia or other blood diseases that involve their immune systems are very susceptible to hospital-acquired infections. Treatment with radiation or drug therapy further reduces the efficiency of these patients' immune systems.
   b. Patients with diabetes, often as a result of the secondary effects of their disease, such as renal insufficiency and acidosis, are very susceptible to nosocomial infections. Diabetic patients who take insulin have more frequent staphylococcal infections than do nondiabetics.
3. Immunosuppressive drugs as a factor
   Patients who are treated with immunosuppressive drugs that suppress the function of their cellular or humoral immune systems, such as those who have received organ transplants, become extremely vulnerable to nosocomial infections. The three classes of immunosuppressive drugs are the lymphocytolytic agents, such as corticosteroids; the metabolic analogues, such as azathioprine; and alkylating agents, such as nitrogen mustard.
4. Physical trauma as a factor
   Patients who have been exposed to any sort of physical trauma are susceptible to infections. Burn patients are especially susceptible to nosocomial infections, especially from *Pseudomonas aeruginosa* and *S. aureus,* organisms that are present in most areas of the hospital.
5. Surgical procedure as a factor
   A surgical procedure in and of itself breaks through one factor in the patient's immuno-defense system. The cutting of tissue breaches a major defense against infection, the skin. Most postoperative infections occur when the alimentary, respiratory, or genitourinary tracts are operated on. The use of anesthesia further affects the patient's defense systems and the prophylactic use of antibiotics also increases the risk of postoperative infection. Surgical wounds are divided into four classes that relate to the probability of postoperative infection:
   a. Clean wounds do not involve a hollow muscular organ, e.g., the gastrointestinal tract, and no break in aseptic

technique occurred. Clean wounds are the least likely to become infected.

b. Clean, contaminated wounds involve the opening of a hollow muscular organ but with minimal spillage of contents.

c. Contaminated wounds are those in which a hollow muscular organ was opened and gross spillage of contents occurred with acute inflammation but without pus formation.

d. Dirty wounds refer to those that contain pus or involve perforation and are the most likely to become infected.

6. Catheterization as a factor

Catheterization is the most important predisposing factor in nosocomial infections because there are so many opportunities for contamination at this site. This is true of any form of catheterization, urinary, intravenous, or otherwise. Microbes may enter the body as the catheter is inserted or as a result of improper handling of the catheter at any time after it has been inserted.

a. Urinary infections result when urine is allowed to flow back into the patient. Also, bacteria have the ability to attach to the bladder's epithelial cells and to the catheter itself, thus causing debris to collect as well as other bacteria to adhere and contributing to infection. Gram-negative bacteremia can result from urinary infection and is a serious complication that can produce case-fatality rates as high as 30% depending on the underlying disease status of the patient. Women are particularly prone to infections related to urinary catheterization.

b. Vascular indwelling catheters are associated with both local and systemic infections. Systemic septicemia is often caused by organisms from the patient's skin, e.g., *S. aureus, S. epidermis,* and *Candida.* Vascular indwelling catheters can be colonized at the insertion site, the catheter hub, via hematogenous seeding of the catheter and via contaminated intravenous fluids.

7. Bacteria as a factor

In areas of the hospital that have a high prevalence of antimicrobial-resistant bacteria, e.g., intensive-care units, colonization of patients with these bacteria occurs even in those who are not being treated with antimicrobial agents if the patient is in the area long enough and is exposed to patients who are being treated with such agents. Antimicrobial prophylaxis is now recommended for only a limited number of procedures, including valve, open heart, and coronary bypass surgery.

8. Injection as a factor

Hypodermic injection can cause infection if (1) the needles or syringes are contaminated, (2) infectious agents on the skin are displaced into the bloodstream or underlying tissue during injection, and (3) the injected solution is contaminated.

9. Instruments as a factor

Medical instruments used for diagnostic procedures such as cystoscopes, urometers, gastrointestinal fiber-optic endoscopes, and so forth have been implicated as sources of nosocomial infection.

V. Organisms That Frequently Cause Nosocomial Infections

About 80% of nosocomial infections are caused by bacteria, most often by gram-negative bacteria. The dominance of gram-negative infections in the hospital is the result of the large number of antibiotics available that affect these species, resulting in the development of antibiotic-resistant strains. *E. coli** is the most frequently isolated pathogen from all body sites (urinary tract, surgical sites, lungs, and bloodstream) of hospitalized patients.

A. Other major bacterial nosocomial pathogens (in order of frequency of infection) include *S. aureus,** coagulase negative staphylococci, *Enterococcus* species, *Pseudomonas aeruginosa,** *Enterobacter* species,* *Candida albicans,** *Klebsiella pneumonias,** gram-positive anaerobes, and *Proteus mirabilis.**

B. Although bacteria have traditionally been the primary concern in nosocomial infections, in recent years fungi and viruses have become more important, largely as a result of AIDS and the increased use of corticosteroids.

1. *Candida* and *Aspergillus** species are the most frequently identified fungal species in hospital infections that are associated with intravenous catheterization. Aspergillus species in particular cause respiratory tract infections via ventilation systems and other sources.

2. Other fungal nosocomial infections include: Zygomy-cosis,* Cryptococcosis, Trichosporosis, Pseudallescheri-asis,* and Fusarium infections. (*indicates species or diseases that are associated with nosocomial pulmonary infections. See Appendix A.)

C. Viruses that are particularly problematic as causes of nosoco-mial infections include: rubella virus, respiratory syncytial vi-rus, herpes simplex virus, varicella zoster virus, hepatitis A virus, cytomegalovirus, and Epstein-Barr virus.

VI. The Hospital as a Special Environment

There are many factors that result from the nature of the hospital and its functions in the community that cause it to be a place where one is particularly likely to become infected with a pathogen.

A. The Physical Facilities

A hospital is an institution to which most of the people in the community who have been identified as being infected with pathogenic microorganisms are funneled. So, at any given time it is the facility within a community where the most dense population of microorganisms reside. Further, the over-use of antibiotics has caused the development of pathologic microorganisms that are resistant to antimicrobial therapy. Some of these microorganisms have become permanent resi-dents of hospitals and are unique to those facilities. Therefore, people who are in a hospital, patients and staff alike, are ex-posed to more and different microbes than they would be ex-posed to under any other circumstances. For example, as many as 75% of hospital personnel can be described as carri-ers of antimicrobial-resistant *S. aureus*.

1. Rooms

After each patient is discharged or transferred, the patient's room must be disinfected to protect the incoming patient, who often is already susceptible to infection. The level of disinfection necessary is dependent on the infec-tious status of the patient who has vacated the room. The possibility of infection is also why flowers are often banned in intensive-care areas and the rooms of immuno-suppressed patients because vase water contains large con-centrations of potentially pathogenic organisms and decay-ing organic matter that may encourage fungal growth.

2. Water

   Unprotected wet areas in hospitals must be considered contaminated by one or more species of "water bacteria," which includes *P. cepacia, P. aeruginosa, Acinetobacter calcoaceticus, Flavobacterium meningosepticum,* and *Aeromonas hydrophila* species. This means that tap water, drains, sinks, shower heads, ice machines, and so forth should be considered contaminated. Distilled water, even if it has been sterilized, may contain endotoxin.

3. Carpets and floors

   Throughout the hospital, care must be taken to keep the microbial population as low as possible on the floor surfaces. As people walk through the hospital, they bring microbes with them. Pathogenic microorganisms on an employee's or visitors' shoes can be moved from one end of the hospital to another in a matter of minutes. Carpets do not appear any more likely to retain a high microbial population than do uncarpeted floors if they are properly vacuumed and kept dry. But they may present an infection hazard when there is direct contact of patients with carpeting, for example, in pediatric wards, or when patients use wheelchairs.

4. Elevator shafts

   As elevators move in their shafts, they displace a large amount of air. In doing so, air is drawn into and pushed out of the shafts through the doors on every floor that they pass (the Bernoulli effect). This causes any airborne microbes to be spread passively from one floor to another.

5. Laundry chutes

   Some of the most heavily contaminated articles in the hospital are removed daily, or more often, from patients and their beds, bundled together, and dropped down chutes throughout the hospital. Hospital laundry is contaminated with every single organic material that human beings can produce. Contact with patients' bed linen is a classic way in which hospital workers contaminate their hands. When patients' linen is bundled together and placed in a laundry chute, the air is displaced just as in an elevator shaft, and air is drawn into the shaft from every section of the hospital. Since some patients' bed linen is changed several times per day, the flow of air following this heavily soiled material is virtually continual. Soiled linen should be removed with as little agitation as possible to reduce the possibility of contamination of the air and the people handling the linen. Soiled or contaminated linen must be bagged, in accordance with individual hospitals' guidelines for the use of specific bag materials, and laundry workers must wear protective gloves and other appropriate personal protective equipment when handling contaminated laundry. The use of detergents and very hot water, 71°C for 25 minutes, to wash linen is essential for the health of the entire hospital population.

6. Food preparation

Because of the susceptibility of hospitalized patients to infection, special care must be taken to ensure that food-borne transmission of disease does not occur. The two most important factors in preventing bacterial food-borne disease are: holding food at correct temperatures, that is, above 60°C or below 7°C, and avoiding cross contamination of cooked food by raw food or by food-handling personnel who have infections. Stuffings and dressings must not be cooked with poultry, especially not within the poultry body cavity. Cooked meat must reach an internal temperature of 74°C as measured by a bayonet-type thermometer. Cooked foods can be kept at room temperature for only minimal amounts of time, and refrigerated food kept at 7°C. Food should be no more than 4 inches deep when packaged for storage. Careful cleaning and decontamination of utensils and surfaces are also vital. Dishes must be washed and rinsed at 82°C for 10 seconds.

7. Ventilation systems

Effective ventilation of hospitals is difficult. The air in hospitals must be moved rapidly enough to reduce airborne contaminants and odors, yet the temperatures must be in a range comfortable for the patients who are attired in gowns or pajamas.

a. Critical-care areas

Critical-care and operating-room areas need to be ventilated at greater rates than for general hospital rooms because the density of patients and personnel is higher in those areas. Coronary-care units should be kept in a narrow temperature range to avoid stress on the patients that can be caused by either hot or cold environments.

b. Nurseries

Newborn infants are very susceptible to infection and the air in nurseries should be moved more rapidly than in general rooms.

c. Burn rooms

Patients with extensive burns, especially those with burns of the upper airways, are uniquely susceptible to infections. Filtered, laminar flow (without turbulence) ventilation for each bed is highly desirable in burn rooms.

d. Air filtration

Filters that ionize microscopic airborne contaminants and/or incorporate high efficiency particulate air filters (HEPA filters) are desirable when they are placed in the ventilation system so that air entering critical-care areas, nurseries, and especially burn rooms is filtered.

e. Negative pressure rooms

The Centers for Disease Control has recommended that patients with active pulmonary tuberculosis and patients receiving aerosolized pentamidine treatments be placed in single patient rooms that have a negative air pressure relative to adjacent areas and are exhausted 100% to the outside of the building.

B. The People

1. Patients are often the sources of nosocomial infections as well as the victims. A great number of patients are admitted to the hospital precisely because they are infected with contagious diseases. Those who are admitted for other reasons often are in the carrier state of undetected infection. All patients bring their normal flora into the hospital, which may include organisms potentially harmful to other patients, especially those who are immunosuppressed.

2. Visitors may be infected prior to their hospital visit with any undetected virulent microorganism, but in any case they carry their personal microbic flora into the hospital. In addition, they may come to the hospital even when they know that they are actively infected. Visitors with upper-respiratory infections frequently do not hesitate to visit a hospitalized friend or relative unless they are counseled by hospital staff

not to do so. Children under age 12 should not be allowed to visit hospital patients. Visitors should not be permitted in the operating or recovery rooms. Visitors in delivery or birthing rooms and intensive-care units should be carefully controlled. The psychological benefits of parents staying in the hospital with their children, however, outweigh concern over the possibility of creating problems of infection.

3. Clearly hospital personnel, because their function is to treat patients, are the most important factor in the spread of infection within the hospital, and there is a real possibility that they may carry infections home. Hospital personnel have several responsibilities resulting from their roles in the overall infection control program.

   a. Personnel must strictly follow approved hand washing procedures. Hand washing is the most important factor in substantially reducing the spread of infection by health care workers (see Chap. 5, IV).

   b. Personnel must follow the infection control procedures developed by the institutions in which they are employed, as well as procedures developed by the specific department or unit to which they are assigned.

   c. Personnel must follow procedures for reporting any needle-stick/penetrating injuries and blood or secretions splash incidents in which they are involved to their supervisor after taking the recommended steps immediately following the incident, e.g., first-aid measures and changing contaminated clothing.

   d. Personnel are responsible for reporting any exposure to or symptoms of infectious diseases to which they have been exposed, in the hospital, in the community, or at home, to their supervisors, so that they may be evaluated by the personnel health service. Examples of symptoms that should be reported are sore throat, skin lesions, productive cough, fever over 100°F, and acute diarrhea.

   e. Personnel should be immunized as recommended by the Immunization Practices Advisory Committee (ACIP) of the United States Public Health Service. As well, prophylactic treatment for exposure to various diseases (see VII, E, 2) is vital for the protection of the patients, health care workers, and their family members.

    f. Personnel do not need to be subjected to routine pro-
grams designed to detect carriers of pathogens, since
such programs are generally not considered to be worth-
while and are, therefore, not recommended.

VII. Hospital Responsibility

Hospitals are responsible for taking every reasonable measure
to reduce the possibility of patients' acquiring nosocomial infections. The Joint Commission on Accreditation of Healthcare Organizations (Joint Commission) holds hospitals responsible on a
professional level. Hospitals are also subject to the authority of
their state public-health agencies. The Centers for Disease Control
in Atlanta, Georgia, performs testing services and provides guidelines for procedures as well as information on infectious diseases
to hospitals.

A. Infections Committee

    The Joint Commission has mandated that each hospital
must establish a multidisciplinary infections committee that
includes members of the medical staff, the administration, the
microbiology laboratory, and the nursing service. Such a committee has numerous responsibilities.

    1. Committee membership

        In practice, the committee membership often includes a
physician chairperson, a hospital epidemiologist; physician
representatives from medicine, surgery, pediatrics, and ob-
stetrics/gynecology; employee health service; a microbiolo-
gist; representatives from the administration and the nursing
service; as well as other appropriate members, e.g., representatives of the blood bank, central supply, or dentistry.

    2. Responsibilities

        The Infection Surveillance Subcommittee, which forms
proposals and makes recommendations to the committee,
reviews departmental infection-control policies and procedures, and assists in complying with Joint Commission
mandates and Occupational Health and Safety Administration (OSHA) standards.

B. Infection Control Team or Infection Control Nurse

    The infection control personnel are responsible for the sur-
veillance of hospital infections, the investigation of clusters or

outbreaks of infection, the development of isolation/precaution policies, educational activities, and reporting notifiable diseases to state divisions of public health.

C. Infection Control Program

An Infection Control Program is basically composed of surveillance, reports, and education.

1. Surveillance of nosocomial infections basically involves the examination of microbiology culture reports, examining of unit records, and communications with medical staff and hospital personnel. Although there is no universal surveillance system, two reporting forms are nearly universal.

a. The infection control nurse fills in a daily work sheet.

b. Report of nosocomial infections contains a summary of the data collected on the daily work sheets. The summary is usually done on a monthly basis.

c. Statistics regarding infection are kept in accordance with standards established by the Centers for Disease Control.

2. Diseases defined as reportable to state departments of public health are reported.

3. Education of hospital personnel takes place through new-employee orientation programs, annual in-service programs, individual instruction, and other methods as appropriate.

4. Consultation with medical staff and employees takes place as appropriate.

D. Physical Facilities and Supplies

Hospitals are required by OSHA standards to provide physical facilities such as readily accessible hand washing facilities and containers for contaminated needles and other sharps, as well as supplies such as appropriate gloves, masks, and gowns for employee use.

E. Employee Health Service

This service, which must be provided at all hospitals, is responsible for protecting the health of both employees and patients. The service functions as part of the overall effort to control the risk of transmission of infections between health care workers and patients. As such, its actions are coordinated with the infection-control program. It contributes to the program through several functions:

1. The service uses placement evaluations to assist in assessing the ability of employees to perform job tasks safely and efficiently. Further, jobs in which employees are placed must not pose unusual risk of infection to the employee, patients, or visitors. The evaluation includes a physical examination, the employee's immunization status, a history of previous medical conditions (such as immunodeficient conditions), and tuberculosis screening.

2. The service is responsible for providing to employees the required immunizations and prophylaxis after exposure to certain diseases. Immunizations include polio; measles (rubeola); mumps; rubella (German measles); tetanus (immunization series or boosters); diphtheria; and hepatitis B vaccine for those who may have exposure to blood or body fluids. Influenza vaccine is recommended on an annual basis for those who are over 65 years of age, those with chronic pulmonary or cardiovascular disease, renal dysfunction, or immunological suppression. Prophylaxis for exposure to hepatitis A, hepatitis B, meningococcal disease, tuberculosis, and rabies should also be offered.

3. The service tests for tuberculosis by the Mantoux (intradermal) method, which is performed initially on all personnel, including volunteers and students, before they are approved to function in the hospital.
   a. Personnel in low-risk areas for contact with active tuberculosis are then tested annually.
   b. Personnel in high-risk areas or departments for contact with active tuberculosis, e.g., emergency room, outpatient services, respiratory care, pulmonary function, microbiology, are tested every 6 months.
   c. Chest X-rays are provided when necessary.

4. The employee health service is responsible for evaluating employees for the presence of communicable diseases, usually when referred by department heads or supervisors, and for determining if those employees should be removed from patient care duties, e.g., those with infectious conjunctivitis or Group A streptococcal disease. Also, infected employees are advised about contact with others, for example, family members.

5. Employee health services are responsible for evaluating any needle-stick/penetrating injuries and blood or secretion splash incidents and taking the appropriate steps to inform and treat affected employees.

6. The service should provide ongoing education to employees on infection control policies and procedures.

F. Department Heads

Department heads, and the supervisors they appoint, have several responsibilities in the overall hospital infection control program.

1. They must follow all recommendations and directives developed by the infections committee.

2. They serve as members of the infections committee or any subcommittee if requested.

3. They develop and maintain, in consultation with the appropriate members of the infections team and departmental medical director, appropriate policies and techniques for patient-care procedures and equipment processing.

4. They provide inservice education on approved techniques and procedures.

5. They provide written, easily accessible policies concerning approved techniques and procedures.

6. They refer personnel with apparent infections such as pink eye, acute diarrhea, sore throat, acute rash, skin lesions or purulent drainage, herpetic whitlow, shingles, productive cough, jaundice, or fever over 100°F, to the personnel health service for evaluation and follow the service's recommendations regarding that evaluation, e.g., reassigning an employee or sending an employee home.

7. They follow hospital procedures regarding the reporting of any needle-stick/penetrating injuries and blood or secretions splash incident involving an employee, and refer the employee to the personnel health department.

SUGGESTED READING

American Academy of Pediatrics and American College of Obstetricians and Gynecologists. *Guidelines for Perinatal Care.* Evanston: American Academy of Pediatrics, 1983.

American Thoracic Society, Centers for Disease Control. "Control of Tuberculosis." *American Review Respiratory Disease* 128 (1983): 336.

Brachman, P. S. "Epidemiology of Nosocomial Infections." In *Hospital Infections,* 3d ed. Edited by J. V. Bennett and P. S. Brachman. Boston: Little, Brown, 1992.

Centers for Disease Control. *Guidelines for the Prevention of TB Transmission in Hospitals.* Atlanta: U.S. Department of Health and Human Services (HHS pub. no. [CDC] 82–8371), 1982.

Centers for Disease Control. *Guidelines for the Prevention and Control of Nosocomial Infection: Guidelines for Handwashing and Hospital Environmental Control.* Atlanta: CDC, 1985.

Centers for Disease Control. "Nosocomial Transmission of Multidrug-Resistant Tuberculosis among HIV-Infected Persons—Florida and New York." *Morbidity and Mortality Weekly Report* 40 (1991): 585.

Centers for Disease Control. "Prevention and Control of Influenza: Recommendations of the Immunization Practices Advisory Committee (ACIP)." *Morbidity and Mortality Weekly Report* 39, no. R R-1 (1990): 1.

Goldman, D., et al. "Control of Hospital-Acquired Infections." In *Infectious Diseases in Medicine and Surgery.* Philadelphia: Saunders, 1992.

Goldman, D. A. "Epidemiology of Staphylococcus Aureus and Group A Streptococci." In *Hospital Infections,* 3d ed. Edited by J. V. Bennett and P. S. Brachman. Boston: Little, Brown, 1992.

Haley, R. W., et al. "Surveillance of Nosocomial Infections." In *Hospital Infections,* 3d ed. Edited by J. V. Bennett and P. S. Brachman. Boston: Little, Brown, 1992.

Hoeprich, P. D., M. C. Jordan, and A. R. Ronald. *Infectious Diseases,* 5th ed. Philadelphia: J. B. Lippincott, 1994.

Jarvis, W., J. R. Edwards, and the National Nosocomial Infection Surveillance (NNIS) System. "Nosocomial Infection Rates in Adult and Pediatric Intensive Care Units in the United States." *American Journal of Medicine* 91 (1991): 3B.

Jarvis, W. R., and W. J. Martone. "Predominant Pathogens in Hospital Infections." *Journal of Antimicrobial Chemotherapy,* 29, suppl. B (1991): 65.

Joint Commission on Accreditation of Healthcare Organizations. *Accreditation Manual for Hospitals.* Chicago: Joint Commission, 1992.

Nelson, J. D. "The Newborn Nursery." In *Hospital Infections,* 3d ed. Edited by J. V. Bennett and P. S. Brachman. Boston: Little, Brown, 1992.

Pittet, D., L. A. Herwaldt, and R. M. Massanari. "The Intensive Care Unit." In *Hospital Infections,* 3d ed. Edited by J. V. Bennett and P. S. Brachman. Boston: Little, Brown, 1992.

Polder, J. A., O. C. Tablan, and W. W. Williams. "Personnel Health Services." In *Hospital Infections,* 3d ed. Edited by J. V. Bennett and P. S. Brachman. Boston: Little, Brown, 1992.

Pugliese, G., and C. A. Hunstinger. "Central Services, Linens and Laundry." In *Hospital Infections,* 3d ed. Edited by J. V. Bennett and P. S. Brachman. Boston: Little, Brown, 1992.

Rahame, F. S. "The Inanimate Environment." In *Hospital Infections,* 3d ed. Edited by J. V. Bennett and P. S. Brachman. Boston: Little, Brown, 1992.

Simmons, B. P., and E. S. Wong. "Guidelines for Prevention of Nosocomial Pneumonia." *Infection Control* 3 (1982): 327.

Villarino, M. E., et al. "Foodborne Disease Prevention in Health Care Facilities." In *Hospital Infections,* 3d ed. Edited by J. V. Bennett and P. S. Brachman. Boston: Little, Brown, 1992.

Chapter 3

Review of Medical Microbiology

CHAPTER OBJECTIVES

Upon completion of this chapter, the reader will be able to

Bacteria

1. discuss the two basic relationships that human beings have with microorganisms
2. compare and contrast the structures of prokaryotes, eukaryotes, and viruses
3. describe the differences between the cell walls of gram-positive and gram-negative bacteria
4. discuss the importance of sporulation
5. compare and contrast the oxygen requirements of obligate aerobes, microaerophiles, facultative anaerobes, and obligate anaerobes
6. contrast the concepts of intoxication (caused by neurotoxins) and infection
7. describe the principle behind the use of hyperbaric oxygen therapy in the treatment of gas gangrene
8. discuss the reasons why mycobacteria can be described as different from most gram-negative and gram-positive bacteria

Viruses

1. compare and contrast viral replication with bacterial replication
2. describe the three types of vaccines

3. discuss how Reye's syndrome can become a complication of influenza and/or varicella-zoster infections

4. discuss the reason that respiratory syncytial virus is the major cause of lower respiratory infections in infants and young children

5. describe how zoonoses like hemorrhagic fevers are transmitted to human beings

6. describe the two modes of transmission through which children acquire human immunodeficiency virus (HIV) infections

7. discuss the groups for which hepatitis B vaccine is recommended and why it is recommended for each group

Fungi

1. discuss the groups that most often experience serious fungal infections

2. compare and contrast the characteristics of yeasts and molds

3. discuss the reasons for the increase in the number of *Candida* infections in recent years

4. discuss the reasons that systemic fungal infections are difficult to treat

5. describe the three manifestations of allergic aspergillosis

Parasites

1. discuss the concept of intermediate host

2. describe the life cycle of *Ascaris lumbricoides*

3. discuss the reason that pork products should be cooked thoroughly

4. list the general categories of disease that are spread by arthropods

I. Relationships between Human Beings and Microorganisms

Many microorganisms inhabit the human body throughout its lifetime. These include both bacteria and fungi. At birth, human beings acquire microorganisms from both the mother and others with whom they come into contact. Specific microorganisms establish themselves, or colonize, specific areas in the body and are called microflora. The most important body sites that are colonized are the upper-respiratory tract, the lower-intestinal tract, and the skin. The blood, spinal fluid, and urine are normally sterile. An individual's microflora stays with that person, or host, for life with minor changes occurring as the result of disease, dietary alterations, or hormonal changes. Microorganisms in the host can have two kinds of relationships with the host.

A. Commensalism

Microorganisms that benefit from their relationship with the host without causing harm are referred to as commensals.

B. Parasitism

Microorganisms that benefit from their relationship with the host at the expense of the host are referred to as parasitic. Commensals can act as parasites if the host's defenses become compromised by things such as age, acquired HIV, poor nutrition, and burns. Parasitism may or may not actually damage the host. There are two types of parasites.

1. Extracellular parasites attach to the surface of host tissue and may produce toxins that enable them to colonize and damage tissue. Diseases caused by extracellular parasites usually produce symptoms for only a short period.

2. Intracellular parasites, especially viruses, live within host cells. There are two types of intracellular parasites.

a. Facultative intracellular parasites can live either inside or outside host cells.

b. Obligate intracellular parasites can replicate only inside host cells. These parasites, except viruses, usually produce diseases that are chronic, or long lasting.

II. Cell Types (Figure 3-1)

Microorganisms can be classified according to their physical characteristics.

A. Prokaryotic (from the Greek *protos,* primitive, and *karyon,* nucleus)

1. Prokaryotes average 1–3 μm in length, have cell walls and a cytoplasmic membrane, and smaller ribosomes but no nuclear membrane or nucleolus. Reproduction is asexual, accomplished through binary fission.

Hereditary information is contained in DNA, via a single chromosome. Respiration is associated with particles in the cytoplasmic membrane.

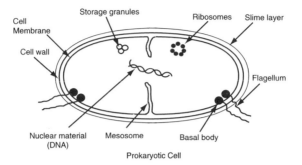

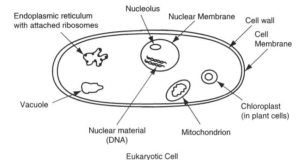

Figure 3–1 The Structural Differences between Eukaryotic and Prokaryotic Cells.

    2. Prokaryotes are found in environments that may or may not contain oxygen, and some require a living host in order to reproduce.

    3. Bacteria are prokaryotes.

  B. Eukaryotic (from the Greek *eu,* true, and *karyon,* nucleus)

    Eukaryotes average 5–10 μm in length (fungi and algae have cell walls), a cytoplasmic membrane, and larger ribosomes, nuclear membranes, and a nucleolus. Reproduction can be both sexual and asexual. Hereditary information is contained in DNA via more than one chromosome.

  C. Virus

    These organisms were originally thought to be small bacteria. Viruses can infect bacteria.

1. Viruses average 20–300 μm in length. They do not have a cell wall, a true cytoplasmic membrane, nucleolus, or ribosomes. They reproduce asexually. Hereditary information can be contained in either DNA or RNA, and may be single- or double-stranded.
2. Viruses can reproduce only within living organisms.

III. Bacterial Structure

A. Size

Bacteria range in length from 0.2–60 μm, but most of those that cause human disease are 1–3 μm long. Since the length of a bacterium varies depending on its stage of growth and environmental factors, size is not considered to be a useful means of classification.

B. Shape (Figure 3–2)

Bacteria are grouped according to four basic shapes.

1. Cocci (singular, coccus) are spherical in shape. When cocci divide they often remain attached and form different groupings.

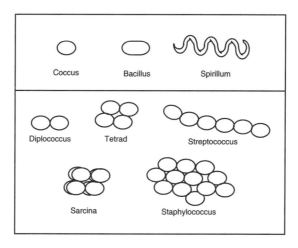

Figure 3–2 Bacterial Morphology. *Top,* Shapes of Bacteria. *Bottom,* Arrangements of the Cocci.

    a. A pair of cocci are called diplococci.
    b. A chain of 4 to 20 cocci are called streptococci.
    c. Cocci that divide in two planes are a tetrad.
    d. Division in three planes results in a group of eight, called a sarcina; if they form large clusters, they are called staphylococci.
  2. Bacilli (singular, bacillus) are rod-shaped bacteria that usually appear singly. The term *bacillus,* which refers to a bacterial shape, should not be confused with the bacterial genus named *Bacillus.* Some bacilli are oval and resemble both coccus and rod shapes. They are called coccobacilli.
  3. Spiral-shaped microorganisms are either helical or corkscrew in shape.
  4. Square-shaped bacteria are not known to be infectious.
C. Pleomorphism
  Pleomorphism is the existence of different forms of the same species or strain of bacterium, usually in its natural environment.
D. Cytoplasmic Membrane
  The cytoplasmic membrane surrounds the cytoplasm of the cell and is involved in several cell functions including:
  • passive diffusion
  • facilitated diffusion (involving carrier proteins)
  • active transport (the most important function)
  • group translocation, which is similar to active transport
E. The Cell Wall
  The bacterial cell wall is a thick, somewhat rigid, layer outside the cytoplasmic membrane that protects the membrane and gives shape to the bacterium. Cell walls, with a few exceptions, are classified according to their reaction to a test called Gram's stain (see Chap 8).
  1. Gram-positive bacteria
    Gram-positive cell walls stain blue or violet. The peptidoglycan layer of a gram-positive cell wall is much thicker than a gram-negative cell wall and contains teichoic acid.
  2. Gram-negative bacteria
    Gram-negative cell walls are multilayered, having an outer membrane covering the peptidoglycan layer, and have protein channels called porions.

3. Cells without walls
   a. Some artificially altered cells can exist without cell walls. A protoplast has no cell wall, and is produced from a gram-positive cell. A spheroplast retains some amount of cell wall and is produced from a gram-negative cell.
   b. The genus *Mycoplasma* does not have a cell wall.
   c. An L-form is a bacterial variant without a cell wall. These bacterial forms sometimes occur spontaneously or may be induced by penicillin or ultraviolet light. Some are stable, but some can revert to their normal state.
F. Capsules and Slime Layers
   Bacterial cells may possess substances called extracellular polymeric substances (EPS) that attach externally to their cell walls.
   1. Capsules are EPS that have some organization and are strongly attached to the cell wall.
   2. Slime layers are EPS that are more loosely organized and are not strongly attached to the cell wall.
   3. EPS are not necessary for the survival of the cell but when present perform the following functions:
      • EPS enable microorganisms to adhere to surfaces or to other microorganisms
      • EPS assist some bacteria in resisting phagocytosis
      • The EPS of some bacteria are antigenic

IV. **Bacterial Movement**

Many bacteria are capable of independent and directional movement, made possible by appendages.
A. Flagella are protein appendages, up to 20 µm long. They are not necessary for the survival of a cell but they enable it to move in response to stimuli toward favorable environments and away from unfavorable environments. Such movement is called taxis. Factors that influence movement include light (phototaxis), air (aerotaxis), and nutrients (chemotaxis). Flagella are arranged in four different patterns.
   1. Monotrichous bacteria have a single flagellum at one pole of the cell.
   2. Lophotrichous bacteria have a tuft of flagella at one pole.
   3. Peritrichous bacteria are covered with flagella.

4. Amphitrichous bacteria have one flagellum at each pole of the cell.
B. Axial filaments are similar to flagella but are located beneath the outer surface of the cell. They are found on spirochetes and enable spirochetes to move through viscous material more easily than do bacteria with flagella.
C. Pili (singular, pilus), like flagella, are protein appendages but are much shorter. They are often referred to as fimbriae. There are two types of pili.
   1. Sex pili range between one to three in number and facilitate the transfer of DNA between donor and recipient cells in a process referred to as conjugation. This is a process of genetic transfer that is used primarily by gram-negative cells, but some gram-positive species use it also. In conjugation the donor cell is called the F+ cell, and the recipient cell is called the F- cell.
   2. Attachment, or common, pili are much more numerous and are used to attach the cell to surfaces. These pili are found most often on gram-negative bacteria and can be important in the disease process.

V. Structures within the Cell

Many bacteria can store chemical compounds and various inclusions within their cytoplasm. In addition, several structures may be found within the cytoplasm.
A. Nucleoids are areas of DNA concentration involved in cell division. Between one and four nucleoids can be present depending on the rapidity of cell division.
B. Ribosomes are composed of approximately 60% RNA and 40% protein and are involved in protein synthesis.
C. Inclusion bodies are particles found within a cell's cytoplasm. In bacteria that infect human beings, glycogen, lipid, and polyphosphate granules are found. Gas vacuoles, polyhedral bodies, and sulphur granules are found in other bacteria.
D. Endospores such as some active (vegetative) gram-negative bacteria can, under unfavorable growth conditions such as depleted nutrients or lowered oxygen tension, cease vegetative growth and produce endospores via the sporulation process.
   1. The sporulation process begins with the DNA being extended along the length of the cell.

2. Then the cell membrane invaginates, compartmentalizing the DNA, and a second membrane forms. The unit is referred to as a forespore.
3. A cortex then forms around the unit and a coat of peptides impermeable to water develops.
4. The vegetative portion of the cell disintegrates and the spore is released into the environment.
5. Spores are very resistant to chemical and physical agents. Temperatures of 121°C for at least 15 minutes at 15 pounds per square inch pressure are required to ensure the destruction of most heat-resistant spores.
6. Examples of bacteria that form spores are *Bacillus anthracis, Bacillus cereus, Clostridium botulinum, C. tetani,* and *C. perfringens.*
7. Spores are able to transform into vegetative cells even after hundreds of years if activated by changed environmental conditions.

VI. Bacterial Reproduction and Growth

Bacterial cells reproduce by increasing their cellular constituents and then dividing.
A. Bacterial Cell Division
   Bacterial cells reproduce asexually by dividing in a process called binary fission which produces two cells, sometimes called daughter cells. Each cell contains the same amount and kind of DNA as the original cell. The process takes place in three steps.
   1. New cell-wall material grows inward from the two sides of the cell.
   2. As the new wall grows, the cell material is divided.
   3. The new walls meet with each new cell possessing a molecule of DNA. Cell division is then complete and the cells separate.
B. Bacterial Growth (Figure 3–3)
   Many factors influence the ability of bacteria to grow. In a suitable environment, bacterial growth follows a definite pattern.
   1. The increase in bacteria is geometric. That is, they increase in the pattern of 1, 2, 4, 8, 16, and so forth. The time re-

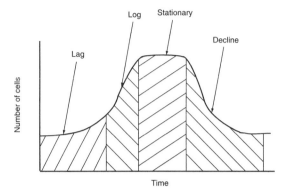

Figure 3–3 The Growth Curve of a Bacterial Culture.

quired for a given cell or a population of cells to divide is called the generation or doubling time.

2. This growth pattern, when plotted graphically, presents a standard curve that shows four distinct phases.

a. The first part of the curve is called the lag phase. In this stage, the cells are adjusting to their environment and are synthesizing biochemicals for future growth. During this phase, the cell population either divides in a nongeometric fashion or does not divide at all, resulting in a nearly horizontal line on the growth curve.

b. The second part of the curve is called the log phase. The term *log* is an abbreviation for the word *logarithmic,* referring to the geometric or logarithmic nature of the cell division. During the log phase, growth occurs at a constant rate and the rate depends on three factors.

(1) Each species' own minimum and maximum growth rate determines growth.

(2) Higher concentrations of nutrients promote growth.

(3) Increases in temperature, up to specific limits, accelerate growth.

c. The third part of the curve is called the stationary phase. This begins as the available nutrients are depleted and the number of dying cells is approximately the same as those still dividing. Other changes that cause the slowing of growth are

- a reduction of pH in the environment
- an accumulation of toxic waste products
- a reduction of available oxygen
- physical and chemical changes occur at this stage that can cause the formation of spores in bacteria, e.g., *Bacillus* and *Clostridium.*

   d. The final part of the curve is called the death and decline phase. This is basically the reverse of the exponential part of the curve. In this phase, cells die in a geometric fashion as a result of accumulated toxic waste products.

VII. Chemical Requirements for Bacterial Growth

Chemicals that are necessary for microbial growth are called nutrients, and they may be organic, inorganic, or a combination of both.

A. Water is necessary for the breakdown of certain compounds and facilitates their transport across the cell membrane.

B. Carbon is required for growth by all microorganisms. Most must be supplied with carbon in an organic form. Such organisms are called heterotrophs.

C. Nitrogen is utilized by most microorganisms in inorganic form, such as ammonia (NH_3). Some microbial forms can use nitrogen gas (N_2). These organisms are found in soil and water. They utilize nitrogen gas in a process called nitrogen fixation.

D. Sulphur is necessary for the formation of some amino acids.

E. Phosphorus is important in the synthesis of DNA and RNA.

F. Minerals are needed by microorganisms, but the need varies greatly. Some of the most frequently utilized minerals are calcium, cobalt, iron, magnesium, manganese, molybdenum, potassium, sodium, and zinc.

G. Vitamins are also needed by microorganisms in varying amounts. Some of the most frequently used vitamins are thiamine, riboflavin, and niacin.

H. Oxygen is very important for microbial metabolism, and oxygen use provides a method of microbial classification.

   1. Obligate aerobes are totally dependent on oxygen for growth. They require an oxygen concentration of 20%, or 0.2 F_{IO_2}, in order to grow, and they can tolerate high environmental concentrations of oxygen.

   2. Microaerophiles are also dependent on oxygen for growth but can only tolerate 4 percent or 0.04 F_{IO_2}.

3. Facultative anaerobes grow best under aerobic conditions, but can alter their metabolism to grow in the absence of oxygen.
4. Obligate anaerobes can grow only in the absence of oxygen. Generally obligate anaerobes are found in the soil but some are found in the intestinal tract and the gums of human beings. Some obligate anaerobes cannot tolerate any oxygen at all; but others, called aerotolerant, can grow in the presence of oxygen.

VIII. **Physical Requirements for Microbial Growth**

A. Hydrogen Ion Concentration
The growth of microorganisms is affected, to a large extent, by the hydrogen ion concentration (pH) in their environment.
1. Most bacteria grow best in a pH range of 6 to 8. Because the pH in the human stomach is approximately 2, most microorganisms are unable to cause infections in the stomach.
2. Fungi grow most rapidly in a pH range between 5 and 6.

B. Temperature
Microorganisms in general can survive in the temperature range of $-10°C$ to $90°C$. They are classified by the temperature range in which they grow best.
1. Psychrophiles have a temperature range for optimal growth between $-10°C$ and $20°C$. Psychrophiles sometimes contaminate food and dairy products; thus refrigeration can actually stimulate their growth.
2. Mesophiles grow best in a temperature range between $30°C$ and $37°C$. Most microorganisms that cause human disease are mesophiles.
3. Thermophiles grow optimally in a range between $45°C$ and $70°C$. They are usually not causes of human disease.

C. Osmotic Pressure
Exposure to highly ionic solutions causes cells to lose water from their cytoplasm, which results in cell shrinkage that is called plasmolysis. Plasmolysis prevents cell growth. Solutions high in either salt or sucrose cause cells to lose water and are used in curing meats.

D. Radiation
Light is required for some bacteria to grow, but some forms of light have destructive effects.

1. Ultraviolet wavelengths are bactericidal.
2. X-rays and gamma rays are also lethal to bacteria.

IX. Chemotherapy

A. Chemotherapeutic agents are compounds used to treat disease.
   1. The two most general categories of chemotherapeutic agents are
      a. Synthetic compounds, which are produced chemically.
      b. Antibiotics, which are produced biologically by microorganisms. Compounds that are produced biologically and then altered by the addition of chemicals are referred to as semisynthetic drugs.
   2. The antimicrobial potential of a chemotherapeutic agent may be
      a. Broad spectrum, that is, active against both gram-positive and gram-negative species.
      b. Narrow spectrum, or active against only one group or even one species of microorganisms.
B. Chemotherapeutic agents are either bactericidal or bacteriostatic (see Chap. 4, I, F and G). Bactericidal agents are effective in situations in which infectious agents must be killed quickly. Bacteriostatic agents stop the growth of infectious agents, allowing the host to develop antibodies against that agent.
C. Chemotherapeutic agents are classified according to the mechanism through which they affect the metabolism of infectious agents. (See Appendices B and C.)
   1. Inhibitors of Cell Wall Synthesis
      These drugs are effective only against cells that are actually synthesizing cell walls and are bactericidal.
      a. Penicillins are the least toxic of all drugs used in chemotherapy, but up to 8% of all persons who receive penicillins experience allergic reactions that can include anaphylaxis.
      b. Cephalosporins are similar to penicillins and are often used when a patient is allergic to penicillin or is infected with a penicillin-resistant species. Three generations of cephalosporins have been developed.

      c. Carbapenems include the class imipenem, which is effective in treating infections caused by gram-positive bacteria (except methicillin-resistant staphylococci), many gram-negative cocci and Enterobacteriaceae, and many anaerobes.

      d. Bacitracin is active against gram-positive, but not gram-negative species.

      e. Vancomycin is used in some staphylococcal infections and in the treatment of antibiotic-associated pseudomembranous colitis.

2. Inhibitors of Cytoplasmic Membrane Function

      a. Polyenes are used primarily against fungal infections.

      b. Azoles are broad spectrum antifungal agents.

      c. Polymyxins are used to treat gram-negative bacterial infections.

3. Inhibitors of Protein Synthesis

      a. Aminoglycosides may be either bactericidal or bacteriostatic depending on the type and depth of the infection and are often used in combination with other antimicrobials to treat serious gram-negative infections. Strains of bacteria resistant to aminoglycosides have developed recently.

      b. Tetracyclines are broad spectrum bacteriostatic agents, effective against gram-positive and gram-negative bacteria, rickettsiae, mycoplasmas, spirochetes, chlamydiae, and some protozoa. Long-term use can result in the development of superinfection by indigenous fungi, e.g., *Candida*. Tetracyclines also cause staining of developing teeth in children. They are frequently used to treat upper respiratory diseases.

      c. Chloramphenicol is a broad spectrum bacteriostatic agent, but is very toxic.

      d. Erythromycin belongs to the group called macrolides which are low in toxicity. They are used in infections caused by Chlamydia, Campylobacter, Mycobacterium avium-intracellulare complex, Mycoplasma pneumoniae, and Legionnaires' disease.

      e. Lincomycin and clindamycin are most often used in the treatment of anaerobic pulmonary infections. A side effect of these drugs is pseudomembranous colitis.

f. Spectinomycin is similar to aminoglycoside and is used to treat pediatric gonococcal infections.

4. Inhibitors of Nucleic Acid Synthesis

   a. Rifampin is used in the treatment of mycobacterial and gram-positive species infections. It is used in combination with other antimicrobials in the treatment and prophylaxis of tuberculosis.

   b. Nalidixic Acid and the quinolones are effective against gram-negative species and are used to prevent infections in cancer patients.

   c. Flucytosine is used to treat yeast infections when given with amphotericin B.

   d. Amantadine is used for the prevention of influenza A but is not a substitute for the vaccine.

   e. Ribavirin is used in the treatment of respiratory syncytial virus and Lassa fever virus infection. It is provided in powder form, which is reconstituted and administered via aerosol.

   f. Idoxuridine is used in the treatment of herpes keratitis.

   g. Vidarabine is used in the treatment of herpes simplex virus infections.

   h. Acyclovir is selectively metabolized by virus-infected cells and is used in the treatment of herpes simplex virus infections.

   i. Zidovudine (azidothymidine or AZT) inhibits HIV. While toxic, it prolongs the survival of patients with advanced HIV infection.

5. Antimetabolites

   a. Sulfonamides are bacteriostatic agents used in the treatment of urinary infections and diarrhea caused by *E. coli* infection.

   b. Para-aminosalicylic Acid (PAS) and the Sulfones. PAS was used to treat infection by M. tuberculosis, but has been replaced. Sulfones are used to treat leprosy.

   c. Trimethoprim is used in combination with sulfamethoxazole to treat hospital associated infections caused by gram-negative bacteria and Pneumocystis pneumonia associated with HIV infection.

   d. Ethambutol is used in the treatment of tuberculosis but is effective only against growing microorganisms.

e. Isoniazid is used in combination with other drugs to treat tuberculosis.
f. Nitrofurans exhibit antibacterial, antiprotozoal, and antifungal activity.

X. Bacterial Diseases
A. Gram-Positive Cocci
Important genera of gram-positive cocci are *Staphylococcus, Streptococcus,* and *Enterococcus.* They, along with gram-negative cocci, i.e., *Neisseria,* are often referred to as pyogenic (pus-generating) cocci.

1. The staphylococci
Members of the genera *Staphylococcus* and *Micrococcus* belong to the family Micrococcaceae. The most important species are *S. aureus, S. epidermis,* and *S. saprophyticus.* The latter two are opportunistic or nosocomial pathogens, and *S. aureus* is a pathogen. Staphylococci clump together in groups like grapes. They are aerobic to facultatively anaerobic, nonmotile, and nonsporeforming. Staphylococci are major natural inhabitants of the skin, armpits, anterior nares, and perineum. In lesser numbers, they are found in the throat, mouth, vagina, intestinal tract, and mammary glands.

a. *Staphylococcus aureus* causes serious infections in various areas of the human body.
(1) Skin infections
S. aureus causes many types of skin infections (pyoderma) including abscesses, furuncles, sties, carbuncles, impetigo, and scalded skin syndrome.
(2) Gastrointestinal infections
(a) Staphylococcal enterocolitis is an overgrowth of *Staphylococcus* caused by the use of oral antibiotics and is known as a superinfection.
(b) Staphylococcal food poisoning is caused by Staphylococcal enterotoxin, after the ingestion of contaminated ham, poultry, egg, and potato salads. It causes projectile vomiting, cramping, diarrhea, and prostration but is rarely fatal. Recovery occurs in 24 to 48 hours.

(3) Deep infections

Deep infections may be primary infections, or they may be the result of an infection that has metastasized from a cutaneous infection. They occur primarily in persons with preconditions such as diabetes, burns, cystic fibrosis, or lower respiratory tract infections and may cause endocarditis, meningitis, pneumonia, septicemia, osteomyelitis, and toxic shock syndrome.

(4) Antibiotic resistant

Most strains of *S. aureus* are penicillin resistant. For those strains methicillin, nafcillin, or oxacillin is used. Methicillin-resistant strains are treated with vancomycin and sometimes with rifampin or gentamicin.

(5) Hospital personnel

Hospital personnel with staph lesions should not come into contact with patients. The carrier rate for hospital workers is 70% to 80%, compared to 30% in the general population. Nursery and surgical patients are most susceptible to staphylococcal infections.

b. Coagulase-negative staphylococci, specifically *S. epidermis* and *S. saprophyticus,* cause disease in human beings. *S. epidermis* is frequently the cause of infections associated with synthetic catheters, heart valves, prosthetic hips, and so forth. The ability of *S. epidermis* to adhere to foreign devices is the result of the production of a slime layer. Resulting infections include endocarditis, colonization of prostheses, bacteremia, wound, and urinary infections. *S. saprophyticus* causes urinary infections. Vancomycin is usually the drug of choice for treating infections caused by these organisms.

c. The Micrococci are similar to staphylococci and are found in the soil and in fresh water. They can cause endocarditis.

2. The streptococci

Streptococci are gram-positive facultative anaerobes, although a few are strict anaerobes. They are spherical in shape and appear in chains or clusters.

a. Streptococci are classified in groups A through O. Those groups harmful to human beings are A, B, C, D, and G. Ninety percent of infections in human beings are caused by group A Beta-hemolytic streptococci.

(1) Group A streptococci (*S. pyogenes*) are transmitted from person to person as the result of contact with an asymptomatic carrier who harbors the organism in the upper respiratory tract, skin, or rectum. Food may be contaminated by a carrier. Streptococci diseases are divided into two categories.

   (a) Suppurative (pus-forming) diseases include meningitis, otitis media, pneumonia, puerperal fever, impetigo, cellulitis, and erysipelas.

   (b) Nonsuppurative diseases include scarlet fever, rheumatic fever, acute glomerulonephritis, erythema nodosum, and toxic shocklike syndrome.

   (c) All strains of group A Beta-hemolytic streptococci are susceptible to penicillin G benzathine.

(2) Group B streptococci (*S. agalactiae*) are found in the oral cavity, the intestinal tract, and the vagina of human beings. They often cause disease in neonates, young infants, and postpartum women. They are the most frequent cause of life-threatening disease in newborns.

   (a) Early onset disease is the result of vertical transmission from mother to child in utero or during passage through the birth canal and causes sepsis and pneumonia. The result is a high mortality rate.

   (b) Late onset disease may be acquired from mothers but is believed to occur primarily from contact with the contaminated hands of hospital personnel. Meningitis is a complication of this disease.

   (c) In adults, infection is found in those compromised by diabetes, chemotherapy, or pregnancy, and diseases including endocarditis, meningitis, pneumonia, and postpartum infections.

(d) Group B infections can be treated with penicillin, but ampicillin with or without gentamicin is used for penicillin-resistant strains.

(3) Group C streptococci rarely cause disease in human beings, but one species, *S. equisimilis,* can cause endocarditis, pneumonia, meningitis, epiglottitis, and wound infections. Infections have been associated with the ingestion of unpasteurized milk.

(4) Viridans streptococci are commensals and are present in the oral microflora of human beings. Several species, including *S. anginosus, S. bovis, S. mitis, S. mutans, S. salivarius, S. sangui,* and *S. vestibularis* can cause opportunistic infections including subacute bacterial endocarditis (SBE), which occurs most often in patients with rheumatic fever or congenital heart disease. Penicillin is administered prophylactically to patients with these diseases before and after surgery.

(5) Group D streptococci are commensals in the intestinal tract. Some members have been given the name enterococcus. Enterococci cause infective endocarditis, neonatal meningitis, and urinary-tract infections. Enterococci are the third most reported cause of hospital-associated infections. Treatment is with penicillin or vancomycin plus an aminoglycoside.

(6) Group F streptococci are commensals in the oropharynx and bowels of human beings. They cause cutaneous abscesses that are directly related to trauma. Infections are treated with penicillin.

(7) Group G streptococci cause asymptomatic pharyngitis. Group G strains are found in the pharynx of 20% to 30% of people. Respiratory secretions may be a source of Group G infection.

(8) Anaerobic streptococci are found in the oral cavity, intestinal tract, and the vagina. They cause puerperal sepsis, subacute bacterial endocarditis, and deep-wound abscesses. Infections are treated with bacitracin and chloramphenicol or teicoplanin.

(9) *Streptococcus pneumoniae* (pneumococci) are gram-positive, facultatively anaerobic cocci that

occur singly or as diplococci and inhabit the upper respiratory tract. They are found in 30% to 70% of the population, and only encapsulated strains cause disease. *S. pneumoniae* is the primary cause of community-associated pneumonia and a frequent cause of otitis media. It is the most common cause of bacterial meningitis in adults and the second most common cause of meningitis in children. Infections are acquired endogenously as a result of lowered host resistance. Infection is treated with penicillin G (IV) procaine. Some strains are resistant to penicillin, ampicillin, erythromycin, tetracycline, chloramphenicol, and streptomycin. These strains are treated with vancomycin.

B. Gram-Negative Diplococci
   1. Neisseria species are both pathogens and normal flora in human beings. They are aerobic or facultatively anaerobic, gram-negative diplococci. Where the paired bodies meet, they flatten and appear bean shaped. The pathogenic members grow best in 5% to 10% carbon dioxide.
      a. Neisseria meningitidis (Meningococcus) cause diseases that are divided into three clinical entities:
         (1) Nasopharyngitis is usually asymptomatic but can result in meningitis or septicemia.
         (2) Meningococcal septicemia presents with high fever, arthritis, and rash. Fulminating sepsis can develop, causing necrosis of the adrenal glands. This leads to rapid death. It is believed that meningococcal septicemia may be the most rapidly fatal of all bacterial infections. Destruction of the cortex of the adrenal glands is called Waterhouse-Friderichsen syndrome.
         (3) Meningococcal meningitis in epidemic form results in mental retardation, behavioral defects, and deafness. The mortality rate for this disease is 85%. Human beings are the only natural host for *N. meningitidis*. Spread of the organism is via respiratory droplets.
            (a) Meningococci may be carried in the oropharynx, nasopharynx, and the urinary tract in

adults without causing symptoms. Carriage rates are highest among children. During epidemics, as many as 95% of those tested may be carriers with only 1% developing the disease. A factor in the probability of infection may be the condition of the pharyngeal mucosa and respiratory epithelium because simultaneous viral infection of the respiratory tract seems to be a predisposing factor.

   (b) Treatment of infection is with cefotaxime for children and with cefotaxime plus ampicillin for infants. However, antibiotic therapy is thought to have little effect on mortality.

 b. *Neisseria gonorrhoeae* (*the gonococcus*) infect the cervix, urethra, rectum, oropharynx, and nasopharynx, and may or may not produce symptoms. Gonococcal infections are usually spread by sexual contact, except for conjunctivitis in the newborn and vulvovaginitis in young girls. More than 450 000 cases of gonorrhea are reported to the Centers for Disease Control each year.

   (1) Genitourinary tract infections in the male usually are in the form of acute urethritis, but as many as 40% of infected males are asymptomatic.

   (2) Genitourinary tract infections in females may involve the urethra, Skene's and Bartholin's glands, the endocervix, and the rectum. Since symptoms in these infections are seldom severe, many female patients are unaware of the infection. However, pelvic inflammatory disease (PID) frequently results from infection of the uterus, fallopian tubes, ovaries, and other structures. Approximately 1 million women in the United States experience at least one episode of PID. Three episodes of PID result in a 50% chance of infertility.

   (3) Extragenital infections are of two types.

      (a) Local infections include pharyngitis, conjunctivitis, and proctitis. Blindness in newborns (ophthalmia neonatorum) can result from infection acquired from an infected mother during passage through the birth canal.

(b) Disseminated gonococcal infection results when organisms enter the blood stream and cause fever, chills, myalgia, and malaise. Dermatitis, skin lesions, and arthritis can also develop.

(4) Gonococcal and chlamydial infections frequently coexist, and antibiotic-resistant strains of both have developed. Recommended drug therapy includes ceftriaxone plus doxycycline. Most states require by law that the eyes of newborns be irrigated with a 1% silver nitrate solution (Crede's method) to prevent gonococcal ophthalmia neonatorum. Erythromycin or tetracycline ointments are recommended to act against both gonococcal and chlamydial conjunctivitis.

c. *Acinetobacter* are gram-negative diplococci or coccobacilli found widely in nature and as part of the normal flora of the skin and throat. The species *A. calcoaceticus* is an opportunistic pathogen, especially in hospital-associated infections, including pneumonia, bacteremia, nongonococcal urethritis, meningitis, and wound infections. Infection is treated with gentamicin and penicillin.

d. *Branhamella catarrhalis* is a gram-negative diplococcus that frequently causes maxillary sinusitis and otitis media in children. It can also cause pneumonia, bronchitis, endocarditis, meningitis, conjunctivitis, and septicemia, especially in compromised hosts. Treatment is with erythromycin and rifampin as well as beta-lactams.

e. *Kingella* is a gram-negative coccobacilli that occurs in pairs and short chains. It is sometimes indigenous to the upper respiratory tract and can cause infections in compromised hosts. Infections are treated with penicillin.

f. *Moraxella* are normal inhabitants of the upper respiratory tract and skin of human beings and animals. Associated diseases include pericarditis and pulmonary abscesses, and they are treated with penicillin.

C. Gram-Positive Sporeformers

Bacillus and *Clostridium* are two genera of bacteria that are resistant to heat and many chemical agents. Most species exist as saprophytes, that is, organisms that live on dead or decaying organic matter in the soil, water, or vegetation. Some species do live in the intestinal tract of human beings and animals. Those that are harmful to human beings are quite virulent.

1. *Bacillus anthracis* are nonmotile, facultative anaerobes. Spores are formed only when the cells are cultivated outside animal tissue. *Bacillus anthracis* is the only species of *Bacillus* that forms capsules.

   a. Anthrax, the disease caused by the organism, is actually a disease of sheep, horses, and cattle that is acquired by human beings through inhalation or ingestion of spores. If the bacilli reach the bloodstream, fatal septicemia can result.

   b. Disease in human beings if it is acquired by inhalation is referred to as wool-sorters disease and is an occupational hazard for people who work with livestock or in animal laboratories. The more common form of human disease is cutaneous anthrax, which occurs when the organisms enter the body through abraded skin. Flies and mosquitoes act as vectors for the organism in Africa. Gastrointestinal anthrax results from the ingestion of contaminated meat and is very often fatal, but it is rare in the United States. Throughout the world, epidemics of anthrax are frequent, and control measures include animal vaccination and cremation of infected animals. Human beings can be vaccinated with toxoid.

   c. Treatment of human infection is with penicillin, but streptomycin, tetracycline, and erythromycin are also effective.

   d. *B. cereus* causes many problems

     (1) *B. cereus* causes typical gastroenteritis, which is characterized by diarrhea and abdominal pain.

     (2) It causes gastroenteritis that is characterized by vomiting but not diarrhea.

     (3) *B. cereus* causes nongastrointestinal disease in the hospital (nosocomial infections) via contaminated dressings, intravenous catheters, and linens. It causes ocular disease following trauma to the eye.

     (4) In compromised patients *B. circulans, B. macerans, B. brevis,* and *B. coagulans* can cause infections.

(5) Because bacilli spores are heat resistant, they are used in biological indicators (see Chap. 4, III, D, 2, b). *B. subtilis spores* are used to check the effectiveness of ethylene oxide sterilization. *B. stearothermophilus* spores are used to test autoclave effectiveness, and *B. pumilis* spores are utilized in testing the efficiency of sterilization by radiation.

2. *Clostridium* includes species that live in the water, soil, and vegetation where they play a major role in animal and vegetable putrefaction. They are gram-positive sporeformers. Most species are obligate anaerobes and some are aerotolerant. Most are motile, having peritrichous flagella, except *C. perfringens,* which is nonmotile. Its spores are very heat resistant, able to withstand a temperature of 120°C for up to 15 minutes. Some species are commensals in the mammalian intestinal tract, and a few are pathogenic in human beings.

   a. Diseases caused by clostridia.

      (1) Food poisoning is a noninfectious disease caused by the ingestion of toxin released by clostridia in contaminated foods. *C. botulinum* causes 25% of clostridial food poisoning. *C. perfringens* is responsible for the remainder. Outbreaks of food botulism are usually associated with home-canned food (usually low-acid vegetables and occasionally fish) rather than with commercially prepared food.

      (2) *C. botulinum* produces eight neurotoxins. Type A toxin causes most outbreaks of food poisoning associated with clostridia.

      (3) Botulism resulting from the ingestion of contaminated food is considered to be an intoxication rather than an infection because the illness is caused by the toxin released by the organism rather than the organism itself. The toxin acts specifically on the peripheral nervous system and causes double vision (diplopia) and dizziness often followed by difficulty in swallowing and breathing. Nausea and vomiting may occur. Death can result from paralysis of the diaphragm. The fatality rate for type A poisoning is 75%.

(4) Toxin produced by *C. botulinum* also produces wound botulism. The symptoms are the same as in food poisoning. Again, type A is usually the cause. The fatality rate is 25%. The administration of antibiotics is not effective.

(5) Infant botulism is the most frequently reported kind of botulism. This form of botulism results from the ingestion of spores that release toxin in the intestines. Ingestion of contaminated honey has been implicated in several cases, and honey is not recommended for infants under the age of one. Most affected infants are 6 months old and younger. Infant botulism is being investigated as a cause of sudden infant death syndrome (SIDS).

(6) Treatment of botulism in adults is through the administration of trivalent antitoxin against the toxins of types A, B, and E. The fatality rate for patients with botulism caused by these types has decreased from 60% to 15% over the last 40 years. The reason for the decline is thought to be advances in acute respiratory care.

(7) Gas gangrene is most frequently caused by *C. perfringens* acting together with other species, e.g., *C. novyi, C. septicum,* and *C. histolyticum. C. perfringens* is a nonmotile, aerotolerant organism that produces spores in living tissue. All species that produce gas gangrene are commensals in the intestinal tracts of human beings and animals, and all produce potent toxins. Clostridial toxins that produce disease in human beings are groups A and C.

(a) Gas gangrene develops when spores and vegetative cells enter tissue after trauma, most often in puncture wounds when anaerobic conditions develop at the wound site.

Two types of infection can develop: anaerobic cellulitis, which is not usually severe, and anaerobic myositis or true gas gangrene, which causes delirium, apathy, disorientation, and eventually death, as a result of the effect of the toxins on the vital organs.

Treatment includes the immediate debridement of the wound and the administration of penicillin and tetracyclines. Hyperbaric oxygen therapy is sometimes useful. The principle of this therapy is that 100% oxygen, administered at 3 atmospheres of pressure, produces hydrogen peroxide or superoxide, which are lethal to the organism at the wound site. Oxygen has no effect on circulating toxin.

The risk of gas gangrene's developing as a complication of surgery is a factor when areas of the body that are easily contaminated by microflora are the operating sites. The risk of this type of infection has been greatly reduced since the swabbing of the operative area with iodophors 15 minutes before surgery has become normal practice.

(b) Mild food poisoning, as a result of the ingestion of vegetative type A, *C. perfringens,* is common and associated with meat products. This type of food poisoning is a frequent cause of illness in the United States, and the food vehicles implicated are beef, Mexican food, turkey, ham, and chicken. The principal causes of the disease are inadequate cooking, improper storage, or improper holding temperature. Fatalities are rare. Treatment does not include antibiotics because the disease is not severe and is self-limiting.

(c) Food poisoning associated with *C. perfringens* type C is a serious illness referred to as enteritis necroticans and has a high mortality rate. The illness is a result of ingesting contaminated pork, but it is not usually seen in the United States.

(d) It is believed that *C. perfringens* can cause diarrhea in hospitalized elderly people, even in the absence of a food vehicle.

(8) *C. tetani* causes tetanus, which is an infection associated with traumatized tissue. The organism is found in cultivated soil and in the intestinal tract of about 25% of human beings. In the United States, 48 cases

of tetanus were reported in 1993, but it is a common cause of neonatal death in developing countries.

(a) The complications of tetanus are caused by a neurotoxin called tetanospasmin, which causes continual stimulation of motor neurons in the spinal cord.

(b) The disease can develop as the result of performing ear piercing, circumcisions, and abortions under unhygienic conditions.

(c) A common cause of death in developing countries is tetanus neonatorum, which is the result of cutting the umbilical cord with unsterilized instruments or packing the umbilical stump with mud.

(d) Once *C. tetani* germinate in human tissue and the toxin is released, continued contraction of the muscles occurs and is referred to as tetany. Muscle spasms are seen most often in the jaw and the disease is referred to as lockjaw (trismus), but the disease can occur in any part of the body.

(e) Treatment includes the administration of tetanus antitoxin, penicillin, and the debridement of the wound. Barbiturates are used to sedate the patient and control spasms. Prevention of the disease is attempted through the prophylactic administration of tetanus toxoid with diphtheria, tetanus, and pertussis vaccine (DTP) plus hemophilus influenzae type b vaccine. A booster of toxoid provides protection for 10 to 20 years. If a person does become infected, an additional booster is administered.

(9) *C. difficile* is found frequently in the hospital environment and can cause pseudomembranous colitis in patients being treated with antimicrobials. Vancomycin is used to treat infections. A serious condition in premature babies caused by *C. difficile* is necrotizing enterocolitis, which can lead to shock. Breast-fed babies are not susceptible to this disease.

(10) *C. septicum,* and other *Clostridium* species, can cause serious infections in patients who have leukemia or cancer of the colon.

D. *Corynebacterium Diphtheriae* and Related Bacteria

Corynebacterium is a genus that belongs to a group of bacteria called coryneforms, which are plant and animal pathogens. They are aerobic and anaerobic, nonbranching, gram-positive, nonsporeforming rods.

1. *Corynebacterium diphtheriae* are obligate anaerobic, nonmotile bacilli with a club-shaped appearance. They are found in the upper respiratory tract and on the skin of human beings, who are the organism's natural host.

    a. Diphtheria, the disease caused by the organism, is of two types.

    (1) Respiratory diphtheria is caused by bacilli in the mucous membrane of the oral cavity. Grayish-white exudate, a characteristic of the disease, forms a pseudomembrane over the mouth, pharynx, larynx, or trachea. This results in respiratory obstruction that requires intubation or tracheostomy. If an adequate airway is not maintained, fatalities are caused by the deadly effects of the toxin on the heart tissue.

    (2) Cutaneous diphtheria presents as an impetigolike lesion on the face or legs and is often acquired as the result of insect bites, skin trauma, or poor hygiene. This form of the disease is common in tropical areas but is found in the United States also, primarily in the southern states. Carriers of this form of the disease can also be sources of respiratory diphtheria.

    (3) Prevention of diphtheria is accomplished through prophylactic immunization with diphtheria toxoid. Immunization programs have removed diphtheria from the list of major infectious diseases in the United States, yet epidemics do occasionally occur in limited geographical areas. More than 80% of cases occur in the 1- to 19-year-old age group. In persons who contract the disease and are allergic to the vaccine, penicillin and erythromycin are the treatments of choice. For cutaneous diphtheria, compresses soaked in penicillin are applied to the lesions.

b. Diphtheroids are a group of nonpathogenic corynebac-
teria found in the mouth, vagina, urethra, and on the
skin. This group acts as opportunistic pathogens in compromised patients and causes endocarditis, meningitis,
and osteomyelitis.

c. *Listeria* are nonsporeforming, gram-positive, facultatively anaerobic rods; the most important species is
L. monocytogenes. They are found in the soil, surface
water, plants, sewage, waste milk, and human and animal feces.

   (1) Listeriosis is a rare but serious disease that occurs in
pregnant women, the elderly, and those with immunosuppressive conditions but most often in neonates where it is called neonatal listeriosis. Neonatal listeriosis has two forms.

      (a) Early onset disease is believed to occur in in-
fants who have been infected in utero and is referred to as granulomatosis infantisepticum. It
causes respiratory distress, cyanosis, pneumonia, and apnea. The mortality rate is between
15% and 50%.

      (b) In late onset disease, the infant is infected either
during passage through the birth canal or in the
hospital environment after birth. This disease
causes meningitis. The mortality rate is 10% to
20%.

   (2) The source of infection in listeriosis that is caused
by *L. monocytogenes* is contaminated food, specifically undercooked chicken, soft cheeses, non-
reheated hot dogs, and various foods from delica-
tessens. Usually, persons with underlying illnesses
are most affected.

   (3) Treatment of listeriosis is with penicillin and ampicillin, but prevention of the disease can be accomplished by thoroughly cooking meat, washing raw
vegetables, avoiding raw milk, and washing hands
and implements after handling raw foods.

d. *Erysipelothrix rhusiopathiae* is a gram-positive, facultatively anaerobic, nonsporeforming, rod-shaped bacterium found in decomposing nitrogenous material, animals, fish, shellfish, birds, and swine that are believed

to be reservoirs for the organism. Disease caused by this organism is an occupational hazard for butchers, fishermen, and veterinarians. The organism enters the body via abrasions or puncture wounds, and usually causes a mild infection but can cause systemic disease and thus result in endocarditis. Normally, the illness is a self-limiting one, but if the infection becomes systemic, it is treated with penicillin, cephalosporins, erythromycin, clindamycin, or penicillin G.

E. Gram-Negative Enteric Bacteria

Many gram-negative, nonsporeforming bacilli live as commensals in the intestinal tracts of human beings and animals. Most of these bacilli belong to the family Enterobacteriaceae. The term *coliform* is usually applied to gram-negative, fermentative inhabitants of the intestinal tract, i.e., *Escherichia coli, Klebsiella pneumoniae,* and *Enterobacter aerogenes.* Enteric bacilli are now the major cause of nosocomial diseases, causing septicemia and infections of the urinary and intestinal tracts. Enterobacteriaceae are gram-negative, motile or nonmotile, aerobic or facultatively anaerobic rods, 1–8 μm in length. They may be motile and, if so, are peritrichous. All have pili and can produce capsules.

1. *Escherichia coli* are commensals found in the intestinal tracts of human beings and animals. Some strains, however, are pathogenic and cause extraintestinal as well as intestinal infections.

   a. Extraintestinal infections caused by *E. coli* occur either endogenously when the organism travels from the intestinal tract to the urinary tract, usually outside the hospital environment, or as a result of person-to-person contact inside the hospital. *E. coli* causes about 20% of all urinary tract infections in the hospital. These infections can lead to pyelonephritis.

   b. Intestinal disease can be caused by four groups of *E coli*:

      (1) Enterotoxigenic *E. coli*
      (2) Enteroinvasive *E. coli*
      (3) Enteropathogenic *E. coli*
      (4) Enterohemorrhagic *E. coli* (EHEC)

EHEC produces a Shigalike or Vero toxin. Diarrheal disease from EHEC serotypes, which produces copious bloody diarrheas, is acquired via the ingestion of undercooked hamburger. The serotypes also cause hemolytic-uremic syndrome and thrombotic thrombocytopenic purpura and are associated with hemolytic anemia, renal failure, and thrombocytopenia, which can be fatal. The cause of these entities is ingestion of contaminated meat, in particular, hamburger. Antibiotic therapy is ineffective, so treatment is symptomatic and may include renal dialysis.

(5) Persons planning to travel to areas where sanitary conditions are poor are prophylactically treated with trimethoprim sulfamethoxazole and bismuth subsalicylate. Hand washing prior to handling food and thorough cooking of meat can prevent infections.

2. *Salmonella* are rod shaped, and most are actively motile organisms that can survive being frozen for long periods. The three species are *S. typhi, S. choleraesuis,* and *S. enteritidis.* They cause disease in both human beings and animals.

a. Gastroenteritis is caused by the ingestion of contaminated food or water and causes diarrhea, fever, and abdominal pain for 3 to 5 days.

b. Enteric fever (typhoid, paratyphoid, and nontyphoidal fevers) are caused by serotypes that are more invasive than those that cause gastroenteritis. Enteric fever is characterized by headache, a nonproductive cough, and high fevers and is common in developing countries.

c. Salmonellae can cause bacteremia, which can lead to infection of the bones, cardiovascular system, and the meninges.

d. Infected persons shed salmonellae 5 to 6 months after the acute phase. Carriers are those persons who shed bacilli one year after infection, and most of those are elderly people.

e. Each year, approximately 40 000 cases of salmonellosis are reported in the United States, with fewer than 500 being typhoid fever. The actual incidence of salmonellosis is thought to be close to 1 million. Mortality is highest among children and the elderly.

f. *S. typhi, S. paratyphi A,* and *S. paratyphi B* are harbored only in human beings, and transmission from person to person occurs via fecally contaminated food or water. Contamination of food occurs during the handling of meat and animal products.

g. Nontyphoidal *Salmonella* species are found in many animals such as turkeys, chickens, and swine. Contaminated chicken eggs have caused many outbreaks in recent years. Infections often occur when food is left standing for long periods after preparation.

h. In the hospital environment, the microorganism is spread via the contaminated hands of workers and by fomites. Epidemics have often been reported in nurseries.

i. Treatment of typhoid fever is with third-generation cephalosporins, cefoperazone, and ceftriaxone. Gastroenteritis is not treated with antibiotics. Chronic carriers are administered ampicillin with probenecid, and immunocompromised patients are treated with quinolones.

j. Salmonella infections can be prevented or reduced by proper sanitation measures, careful preparation and refrigeration of food products, and the detection of carriers.

k. Vaccines of *S. typhi* are given to military personnel.

3. *Shigella* cause bacillary dysentery that is transferred by the fecal-oral route. The four species are *S. dysenteriae, S. flexneri, S. boydii,* and *S. sonnei.* Shigellosis is acquired through the ingestion of contaminated food or water, or contact with fomites. Symptoms include abdominal cramps, fever, diarrhea, and dysentery, ranging from mild to severe.

a. The number of cases of shigellosis in the United States is about 25 000 per year, with the highest rates being in children in the western states. Epidemics are often associated with day-care centers, prisons, and other institutional settings.

b. Treatment with antibiotics can shorten the duration of diarrhea, but, since most cases are mild, antibiotics are not usually necessary. The exception is a disease caused by *S. dysenteriae,* which is treated with ampicillin.

c. The incidence of shigellosis can be controlled, or limited, by the use of sanitary measures, by good personal hygiene, and by restricting infected workers from handling food or working with patients.
4. *Yersinia* that are pathogenic are *Y. pestis, Y. pseudotuberculosis,* and *Y. enterocolitica. Yersinia* are normally found only among animals, with human beings being infected almost accidentally.
   a. *Y. pestis* is the agent that causes bubonic (from buboes or enlarged lymph nodes) plague, known as black death. The organism is harbored in rodents and is transmitted to human beings via insect vectors, notably the rat flea. The disease is rarely found today, although it caused a million fatalities in Asia in 1904. In the fourteenth century, it was responsible for the death of 25% of the population of Europe.
   b. Pneumonic plague is caused by the same species and results when the organism is acquired by inhaling the respiratory secretions from an infected person or animal. If untreated, it causes death within 36 to 48 hours.
   c. Plague is usually a disease of rodents. In the United States this includes squirrels, chipmunks, deer mice, wood rats, and prairie dogs. Plague among rodents is called sylvatic plague; when it is transmitted from person to person, it is called demic plague. Treatment is with streptomycin, plus tetracycline or chloramphenicol.
   d. Two species, *Y. enterocolitica* and *Y. pseudotuberculosis,* cause diseases called yersiniosis that affect domestic animals, but human beings can acquire the diseases through the ingestion of contaminated water, milk, and milk products, or through blood transfusions. Infection with *Y. enterocolitica* occurs most often in children and is usually a self-limiting gastroenteritis. Complications, however, can include mesenteric lymphadenitis and reactive arthritis. Antibiotics are not usually administered for gastroenteritis, but doxycycline is given for more serious infections.
5. *Providencia* is the most important cause of severe infection in burn patients, replacing *P. aeruginosa.* It also causes uri-

nary infections. The transmission route is not known, but it is believed to be transmitted via the air. Death as a result of providencia infections usually involves bacteremia or pneumonia. *Providencia* species are very resistant to antibiotics, and treatment relies on special testing performed to identify the organism.

6. *Proteus* is found in soil, water, and the human intestinal tract. Species pathogenic to human beings are *P. mirabilis, P. vulgaris,* and *P. rettgeri.* Proteus infections occurring in hospitals involve the urinary tract, the blood, the soft tissue, and the lower respiratory tract. Infection is most probably spread by the hands of hospital workers. Treatment of infection is the administration of ampicillin, cephalothin, and aminoglycosides.

7. *Klebsiella* commonly infect human beings and are found in the nasopharynx of most adults. Species most frequently found are *K. pneumoniae, K. ozaenae, K. rhinoscleromatis,* and *K. oxytoca.* Hospitalized patients are often colonized by *K. pneumoniae,* which causes septicemia in pediatric wards, and upper respiratory tract infections and bacterial pneumonia in compromised patients. It is actively destructive to lung tissue. Several strains of *K. oxytoca* are resistant to antibiotics. *K. ozaenae* is responsible for infections of the middle ear, urinary tract, and soft tissue, and is thought to be responsible for ozena, which is a chronic rhinitis. Treatment is with aminoglycosides and tetracyclines.

8. *Serratia marcescens* are found quite commonly in soil and water, including hospital preparations of so-called sterile solutions. *S. marcescens* is particularly likely to infect patients who have indwelling catheters and those on antibiotic chemotherapy. Spread of infection occurs through the hands of hospital personnel, and it causes septicemias, infections of the urinary tract, and infections of the central nervous system. Infections are treated with gentamicin, carbenicillin, and kanamycin.

9. *Enterobacter*
   Members of the genus *Enterobacter* are opportunistic bacteria that may cause 4% to 12% of all gram-negative bacteriemia, most of which is hospital acquired.

a. *E. cloacae* is associated with the contamination of intravenous fluids and other hospital equipment. In fact, members of *Enterobacter, Klebsiella,* and *Serratia* genera are the primary cause of contaminated intravenous fluids because they are able to multiply in glucose-containing fluids where most other organisms either die or cannot multiply.

b. *E. aerogenes* and *E. cloacae* are associated with many infections including endocarditis, ventriculitis, and gram-negative meningitis and may be responsible for urinary and lower respiratory tract infections.

c. *E. sakazakii* causes neonatal meningitis and sepsis. The route of transmission is not known.

F. *Pseudomonas* and Related Organisms

   Pseudomads, members of the group to which the genus *Pseudomonas* belongs, are gram-negative, nonfermentative, aerobic bacilli and are opportunistic pathogens normally found in soil and water.

   1. *Pseudomonas aeruginosa* are rod-shaped bacilli. Most are motile and produce slime layers. The organism is unusual because it is biphasic; that is, it can grow in two growth patterns.

      a. It can grow when the organism exists as a highly motile cell.

      b. It can also grow in the form of an adherent microcolony or biofilm as the result of producing a slime layer.

      c. *P. aeruginosa* causes potentially fatal infections in compromised patients, e.g., those with burns, cystic fibrosis, and chronic respiratory disease.

         (1) In patients with cystic fibrosis, *P. aeruginosa* can become the dominant organism in the microflora of the patient's lungs. An unusual morphotype of *P. aeruginosa*—the mucoid morphotype—develops in these patients. The organism produces a biofilm that protects it against phagocytosis and increases its resistance to antibiotics.

         (2) *P. aeruginosa* species is the organism most likely to cause serious infections in burn patients. It is frequently transmitted to these patients via hydro-

therapy involving contaminated water. In fact, water used for recreational purposes, i.e., hot tubs and whirlpool baths, must be kept at a pH of 7.2 to 7.8 in order to reduce the incidence of waterborne infections caused by the organism.

(3) *P. aeruginosa* is also one of the leading causes of gram-negative hospital associated infections in the urinary tract and surgical incisions.

(4) In vitro antibiotic sensitivity tests must be performed before beginning antibiotic therapy, because *P. aeruginosa* strains have developed that are resistant to most antibiotics. Mild infections are treated with polymyxin B, colistin, and gentamicin; more severe infections are treated with carbenicillin plus gentamicin or tobramycin plus azlocillin.

(5) Some other pseudomonads that cause hospital acquired infections are *Acinetobacter* genus, *P. pseudomallei, P. fluorescens, P. cepacia, P. stutzeri, Moraxella* species, and *Flavobacterium* species.

G. *Vibrionaceae*

There are four genera in the family *Vibrionaceae,* but species of the genus *Vibrio* are the most important human pathogens. They are straight or curved rods, gram-negative, motile anaerobes.

1. *Vibrio cholerae* is the cause of Asiatic cholera, which is a gastrointestinal disease that has been a major cause of death for centuries. Although the disease is infrequent in the United States, and those cases have been associated with travel, it is a major cause of illness in developing countries. Cholera can cause the loss of 10 to 25 liters of fluid through vomiting and diarrhea over a period of only a few days. Death results from shock, metabolic acidosis, and renal failure. Even if a person does survive an infection, there is no acquired immunity, and reinfection can occur.

a. Cholera is caused by a strain called *V. cholerae 01,* and is spread via ingestion of contaminated water or food, especially fish. The organism is sensitive to gastric secretions, so a relatively large number of the organisms must be ingested to cause illness. In 1991, an outbreak of cholera began in Peru and spread to most countries in South America, causing more than 4000 deaths.

b. Treatment of cholera basically consists of replacing water and electrolytes intravenously. The solution administered consists of sodium chloride, sodium bicarbonate, and potassium chloride for those patients in severe shock. Antibiotics can reduce the amount of diarrhea significantly. Tetracycline is used for adults, and trimethoprim sulfamethoxazole is given to children and pregnant women.

c. Cholera can be prevented with proper sewage treatment and water purification. Persons traveling to foreign countries, especially Asia and Africa, should not ingest raw seafood or uncooked vegetables. Crabs must be boiled for 10 minutes to assure the death of *V. cholerae 01.*

d. Non-01 *V. cholerae* causes symptoms like those in classic cholera, but they are not as severe. The organisms are found in estuarine waters, more frequently during the warmer months in southern coastal areas. Infection results from ingesting contaminated oysters, mussels, clams, shrimp, and crabs or by drinking contaminated water.

2. *V. parahaemolyticus* is part of the flora of coastal waters and estuaries worldwide. Most infections are associated with the ingestion of improperly cooked crabs and cause abdominal cramps, diarrhea, and vomiting. Severe infections cause dehydration, dysentery, and acidosis. The disease is usually self-limiting, and no deaths have been reported in the United States. The organism can also cause infections of wounds or abrasions if they have been contacted by contaminated water. Treatment is with chloramphenicol, tetracyclines, and aminoglycosides.

3. *V. vulnificus* causes cutaneous infections via seawater where it is part of the normal flora, but it can also be found in fresh water. It can cause septicemia if contaminated raw or undercooked seafood, especially oysters and clams, is ingested. Infections are treated with ampicillin, tetracyclines, and aminoglycosides.

4. *V. alginolyticus* causes ear and other infections, and the illness is the result of swimming in seawater where it is part of the microflora. Treatment involves draining the infected area and administering chloramphenicol, gentamicin, or nalidixic acid.

5. The genus *Aeromonas* normally causes disease in reptiles, amphibians, and fish. They are found in sewage, marine life, and soil. They can cause disease in human beings either through the ingestion of contaminated water or through abrasions. Septicemia can result and is treated with chloramphenicol, gentamicin, and tetracyclines.

6. The *P. shigelloides* species of the genus *Plesiomonas* is found in estuaries and fresh water and causes severe gastroenteritis, which often requires hospitalization. Infection is the result of eating contaminated raw seafood. Infections can cause meningitis, sepsis, cellulitis, and arthritis, but rarely. Treatment is with chloramphenicol, tetracyclines, and aminoglycosides.

H. Gram-Negative Coccobacillary Aerobic Bacteria

This group includes the genera *Hemophilus, Bordetella, Brucella,* and *Francisella.* These organisms are nonmotile and aerobic to microaerophilic.

1. *Hemophilus* are part of the microflora of the respiratory tract. Almost everyone carries one or more species of the genus *H. influenzae,* which causes the most infections. *H. influenzae* is divided into two groups.

a. Encapsulated *H. influenzae,* type b (HIB) infection occurs via inhalation of respiratory droplets from people who are ill, or who are carriers of the organism. After the organism invades the bloodstream, it can cause systemic infections, i.e., meningitis, epiglottitis, cellulitis, septic arthritis, and pneumonia.

(1) HIB strains are the primary cause of bacterial meningitis in children younger than 4 years of age and can cause mental retardation. Adult infections with HIB usually occur in compromised patients and cause pneumonia. Adherence of HIB to the respiratory tract may be the result of impaired mucociliary clearance caused by a viral infection or by smoking.

(2) *H. influenzae* can be cultured from the upper respiratory tract of most healthy people, but 95% of HIB-caused disease occurs in children younger than 4 years of age. Approximately 12 000 cases of HIB infection are reported each year in the United

States. Although the mortality rate is less than 10%, neurological complications occur in 10 to 15% of the survivors. Children in day-care centers are at increased risk of infection. Meningitis caused by *H. influenzae* occurs more often in the fall and spring, and higher rates of infection afflict African-Americans, Native Americans, and Eskimos.

b. Nonencapsulated *H. influenzae* accounts for 75% of the strains normally found in the upper respiratory tract. Pneumonia caused by these strains occurs most often in the elderly and in patients with chronic bronchitis. Further, these strains cause one half of all meningitis cases in adults. In addition, otitis media, sinusitis, bronchitis, alveolitis, conjunctivitis, and infections of the female genital tract are commonly caused by these strains.

c. Many drug-resistant strains of *H. influenzae* have developed, so antibiotic sensitivity tests should be performed before treatment. The administration of sulbactam with ampicillin is the treatment for adults. Cefotaxime and ceftazidime with ampicillin are used for the treatment of meningitis in children. HIB conjugate vaccine is administered with combined DTP vaccines. Rifampin is recommended for any children under two years of age who have had contact with HIB meningitis.

d. *H. ducreyi* causes chancroid, a sexually transmitted disease that is uncommon in the United States but that is prevalent in developing countries. There is a high rate of transmission of HIV between sexual partners who also have chancroid. Chancroid is treated with azithromycin, ceftriaxone, or erythromycin.

2. *Bordetella* are commonly found in the upper respiratory tract of human beings.

a. *B. pertussis* is a strict aerobe that causes whooping cough (pertussis) and is pathogenic only in human beings. It is spread via exposure to aerosols from infected people and causes disease most often in the very young.

b. Pertussis at first presents as a cold, then is characterized by severe coughing that produces the characteristic whooping sound in children (but not usually in adults).

It progresses to blockage of the bronchial tree that can lead to infection of lung tissue by pyogenic (pus-forming) cocci, convulsions, and sometimes death.

c. Treatment of whooping cough is with erythromycin, tetracycline, chloramphenicol, and penicillin to lessen the communicability of the disease and help prevent secondary infections even though the disease is self-limiting. The number of cases of whooping cough has decreased from 120 000 cases in 1950 to 4083 cases in 1992.

3. *Brucella* is a genus of gram-negative, nonmotile *Coccobacillus* that can produce capsules. They are facultative, intracellular parasites that cause disease in human beings and animals.

   a. Brucellosis is a disease acquired by human beings as the result of ingesting raw milk (usually goat's milk), raw-milk products, or meat from infected animals. The disease is unusual in the United States, but travelers are at risk of infection.

      (1) Brucellosis is primarily a zoonosis (a disease of animals transmittable to human beings) and infections occur among farmers, veterinary surgeons, and slaughterhouse workers who have contact with infected animals, particularly swine. Infection in these situations is through the invaded skin or respiratory tract of the hosts. The organisms, after entry, migrate to the lymph nodes, liver, bones, and spleen, where they often become dormant for several months. More often, however, an acute phase occurs within weeks, presenting with a fever, called undulant fever, of between 100°F and 104°F.

      (2) Prevention of the disease is through the proper vaccination of cattle and the slaughter of infected animals. Treatment during the acute stage is with tetracyclines. Chronic infections are treated with doxycycline and rifampin.

4. *Francisella tularensis* is a gram-negative, nonmotile bacillus that can produce a capsule. It is highly pleomorphic (can have more than one shape). *F. tularensis* causes tularemia, a disease of rodents, particularly rabbits, that is transmissible to human beings.

a. Human infection occurs through direct contact with infected animals, handling or ingesting contaminated meat, the bites of insect vectors, or inhaling contaminated aerosols. Most infections are caused by contact with contaminated rabbit tissue during the skinning process (rabbit fever) or from eating contaminated rabbit meat, but one third of cases are the result of the bites of infected ticks or deer flies. Laboratory workers can contract the disease by inhaling aerosols from infected animals. About 250 cases of tularemia are reported each year in the United States.

b. Tularemia usually causes ulceration of the primary lesion, fever, and lymph node swelling but can also affect the spleen, liver, and lungs. The most serious form of the disease is pneumonic tularemia, acquired when contaminated aerosols are inhaled. The fatality rate for this form of the disease can be 30%. Treatment is with streptomycin. An attenuated vaccine is available for use by laboratory personnel.

I. Mycobacteria

Mycobacteria are organisms that can be found in most animals and in human beings. They are different from most gram-negative and gram-positive bacteria because their cell wall is unique, containing a peptidoglycan layer that cannot be stained by gram stain reagents because it resists the acid-alcohol step in the staining process. They can be stained in the Ziehl-Neelsen test (see Chap. 8, I, D, 2 (b)). Mycobacterial cells are also unusual because they divide very slowly, once every 18 to 24 hours, which results in a relatively long time span between infection and the appearance of symptoms as well as a delay in identifying particular species in the laboratory.

1. *M. tuberculosis* and *M. bovis* cause tuberculosis (TB). *M. tuberculosis* is the major cause of TB in human beings in both developed and developing countries; however, *M. bovis* (usually found in cattle) is also a cause of TB in developing countries. TB is a chronic disease in which the TB bacillus usually infects the lungs, though it can infect any body organ. Infection occurs in one of two sequences.

a. As the result of recent acquisition of the disease, a primary lesion develops in the alveoli of one lung. In 3 to

12 weeks, an immunological response occurs and the lesion is walled off in 85% to 95% of infected people, though the lesions still contain viable bacilli. At this stage, no symptoms appear. However, in the remaining 5% to 15% of those who are infected, the bacteria proliferate in the lung or other organs and form tubercles (nodules), which appear as granulomas. The tubercle and most bacilli are then destroyed by the lysosomal enzymes of neutrophils, and the result is a mass of host cells and bacilli, called a caseation (cheeselike) necrosis. This caseous lesion may calcify and contain some viable bacilli. If the lesion later liquefies, a cavity is formed in the lung tissue. The bacilli can also travel through the bloodstream to other organs, to a bronchus, or can be aspirated into the lower areas of both lungs.

b. In reactivation tuberculosis, a TB infection that had seemed to be terminated, the host is reinfected through either activation of bacilli that survived the primary infection or inhalation or ingestion of new bacilli. This type of infection occurs most often in the elderly, but persons suffering from malnutrition or diabetes mellitus, those undergoing steroid therapy, and chronic alcoholics are at increased risk.

c. TB in patients infected with HIV is caused by multidrug-resistant strains of *M. tuberculosis.* HIV-infected persons who have latent TB infections risk active infection at a rate of 7% to 10% per year. In HIV-infected patients who are newly infected, TB develops within 1 to 3 months in 40% of patients exposed to infectious TB patients, and death can result in as little as 6 weeks. TB in patients with advanced HIV infection is often disseminated and may cause infections of the brain or bone, meningitis, gastric tuberculosis, pericarditis, and scrotal TB.

d. Today, TB is a disease affecting primarily older men, alcoholics, drug addicts, and others with depressed immune systems. TB had been considered a disease of infants and young adults some years ago and was considered to be on the decline in the 1980s, but it has steadily increased in incidence recently. Among the factors contributing to this in the United States are increases in homelessness, drug abuse, and poverty; active TB that develops in infected immigrants; and the increase in the number of AIDS cases. In the United States, 10 million people are currently infected with *M. tuberculosis* and 20 000 additional people are infected each year, resulting in about 25 000 new cases of TB each year. Most of these new cases are in people with long-term latent infections.

(1) Tests for hypersensitivity to purified tuberculin protein derivative (PPD) indicate whether an individual has had, or currently has, an infection with the TB bacillus.

   (a) Intracutaneously injected PPD (Mantoux test) in the amount of 5 tuberculin units is the standard test for hypersensitivity. An induration (hardening of tissue) at the site of injection of 1 to 5 mm of PPD, after 48 to 72 hours, is considered to be a negative response. The test is then repeated with a higher dose and, if negative, is presumptive proof that the individual has not had contact with the TB bacillus. An induration of 5 to 9 mm is considered doubtful and the test is repeated. However, an induration of 10 to 33 mm indicates a hypersensitivity resulting from either past or present infection. In patients infected with HIV, an induration of 5 mm or more can indicate TB infection.

   (b) The multiple-puncture method (tine test) of testing for hypersensitivity results in many false positive and negative results and is recommended for use only in large populations in which TB is not prevalent.

(2) Treatment of TB infection is evolving as the epidemiology and drug resistance of the TB bacillus changes. Currently, a 6-month drug regimen is used. For the first 2 months, isoniazid, rifampin, and pyrazinamide are used. For the next 4 months, isoniazid and rifampin are given either daily or weekly. In areas where TB is prevalent, the Centers for Disease Control recommends an initial regimen

of isoniazid, rifampin, and pyrazinamide with other appropriate antibiotics. Patients who are under treatment for TB do not require hospitalization because transmission is not considered to be a factor, as bacilli in secretions that could be aerosolized by coughing or sneezing are destroyed by the medications. Patients with active TB must cover their mouths and noses when sneezing or coughing to prevent the airborne spread of the bacillus.

(3) Multidrug-resistant TB has appeared in institutional settings such as nursing homes and prisons because patients do not comply with prescribed drug-treatment regimens. Some strains are resistant to as many as seven drugs.

(4) Tuberculin skin testing of workers in institutions where there is a risk of TB transmission is important in reducing the spread of the disease. Persons who are infected, but are asymptomatic, are treated with isoniazid. This treatment is also recommended for household members living with patients with diagnosed TB. Treatment is given for 6 months to 1 year. Isoniazid can cause liver damage, so these individuals must be monitored and warned against the hazards of alcohol ingestion.

(5) The bacillus of Calmette and Guérin (BCG) in a live vaccine has been used for the prevention of TB but is no longer recommended for use in adults in the United States because it causes patients to have a positive response to the tuberculin test. Instead, prophylactic administration of isoniazid is recommended. BCG vaccination is recommended for infants and children with negative tuberculin tests who are nevertheless exposed to patients who are untreated, or ineffectively treated, or who have infections resistant to isoniazid and rifampin.

2. Nontuberculous mycobacterioses, referred to as MOTT (Mycobacteria other than *M. tuberculosis*), are different from *M. tuberculosis* in that person-to-person transmission does not usually occur, they can be found nearly anywhere in nature, they are saprophytes, and they can colonize hu-

man beings without causing disease. Infections caused by MOTT are usually invasive only when patients have predisposing conditions but can be problematic in the hospital environment, causing infections following dialysis, open-heart surgery, and insertion of implant devices. MOTT most frequently infect children and immunosuppressed adults. Infection is the result of contact with contaminated food or water. MOTT are very resistant to chlorine and glutaraldehyde.

    a. The complex of *Mycobacterium avium* includes *M. avium* and *M. intracellulare,* which infect patients who have chronic pulmonary disease. Infection becomes systemic and can be fatal if not treated. Infection of AIDS patients with *M. avium* is the most common systemic bacterial infection complicating that disease and contributes to its mortality. The infection begins with a respiratory or intestinal colonization; if the spleen or lungs are then infected, fatality will result. Prophylaxis for the treatment of infection is with rifabutin, charithromycin, and azithromycin. *M. kansasii* also causes serious infections in AIDS patients.

    b. *Mycobacterium fortuitum* complex includes the species *M. fortuitum* and *M. chelonei.* The first species causes cutaneous infections. *M. chelonei* is causative of disease of the skin and lungs, especially in renal-transplant patients and in patients on steroids and cytotoxic drugs and can cause relapsing pulmonary disease.

3. *Mycobacterium leprae* is an intracellular parasite that causes leprosy (Hansen's disease). Transmission of the organism is usually via inhalation of the bacilli. Between 10 and 12 million people have leprosy worldwide, primarily in Asia and Africa. In the United States, there are about 30 new cases per year with most cases appearing in California, Texas, and Hawaii. Transmission is person to person via nasal secretions that enter the host through skin abrasions. *M. leprae* cannot be cultivated in vitro, but only in vivo, on mouse foot pads or armadillos. While a natural infection in armadillos, most human beings have a resistance to the disease, but those who do not and who are exposed develop one of three forms of the disease.

a. Indeterminate leprosy produces hypopigmented areas of the skin and dermatitis, and most people recover spontaneously.

b. Those who do not recover develop lepromatous leprosy, which produces disfiguration through the development of lepromas (nodules) on all parts of the body, predominantly on the face and hands. Most leprosy patients suffer some degree of peripheral nerve damage, leading to a loss of feeling and paralysis of the face, hands, and feet that in turn leads to accidental self-damage and deformity.

c. Tuberculoid leprosy is a localized form of the disease.

d. Treatment is with dapsone and rifampin for 6 months, followed by dapsone for 3 years. Corticosteroids and clofazimine are also used to minimize nerve and eye damage.

J. Spirochetes and Spiral and Curved Rods

Helical and curved bacteria can be found in the soil and water. Some are commensals in animals. A few are pathogenic to human beings.

1. The spirochetes are gram-negative, long, thin, helically shaped cells that are motile by movement of axial filaments at each pole (see IV, B), which enable them to move in a fashion that differentiates them from spiral or curved rods. They are 3 to 500 μm long and 0.20 to 0.75 μm in diameter. Those that are pathogenic to human beings are usually not more than 40 μm long. They can be aerobic, facultatively anaerobic, or anaerobic, and they divide by transverse fission.

a. *Treponema* that are commensals are found in the oral cavity, gastrointestinal tract, and urogenital tracts of animals. Diseases caused by *Treponema* are called treponematosis.

(1) *Treponema pallidum* causes syphilis. This disease is nearly always caused by sexual contact (90%) or accidental contact with infectious lesions. Infection produces several stages of development:

(a) Primary syphilis presents in more than 90% of cases as a single lesion on the cervix of the female or penis of the male. A lesion can also appear on the scrotum, labia, nipples, rectum, eyelids, mouth, or fingers. At the site of initial infection, a lesion called a hard chancre develops about 10 days to 3 months after infection. If untreated, the organism can enter the bloodstream, but in up to 75% of untreated cases the disease does not progress beyond this stage.

(b) Secondary syphilis occurs when the organism moves from the site of primary infection after 6 weeks to several months. More than 80% of those infected develop a rash on the trunk or limbs at this time. Mucous membrane lesions called condylomata can develop around the anus, labia, mouth, tongue, and tonsils. Infected persons are highly infective at both the primary and secondary stages. The ability to infect ends when the lesions heal, but the organism remains viable.

(c) Latent syphilis is the stage in which the viable organisms exist but do not produce symptoms. There are two periods in this stage. Early latent syphilis lasts about 2 years, during which time lesions may reappear and cause the patient to become infective again. The late latent period lasts more than 2 years to a lifetime, during which time the patient is not infective.

(d) Tertiary or late syphilis is the stage that may occur at any time after the primary or secondary stages or may never arise. The noninfective lesions that develop during this stage are called gummas, and they may or may not be debilitating. They do, however, cause ulcerations on the legs, hands, face, and scalp. They sometimes cause bone and cartilage damage. The most serious of these lesions can cause damage to the cardiovascular and central nervous systems. Cardiovascular syphilis is fatal.

(e) Congenital syphilis is contracted by a fetus from a mother who has primary or secondary syphilis if the mother remains untreated before the sixteenth week of pregnancy. Even with treatment, if it is after the sixteenth week, the fetus is at risk of developing bone or joint damage, deafness, or interstitial keratitis. If untreated, 20% to 25% of fetuses die as a result of stillbirth or spontaneous abortion, and 20% to 25% more will die soon after birth. About 50% of those who do survive will have severe infection.

(f) In the United States, the incidence of primary and secondary syphilis increased from 13.7 to 18.4 cases per 100 000 from 1981 to 1989 with 1990 being the highest reported year since 1949. Syphilis in the United States is predominantly a heterosexually transmitted disease, occurring most frequently in the inner cities and among minority populations. The increase in incidence has resulted in an increase in congenital syphilis from 158 in 1983 to 3211 in 1993. It is believed that the major causes of the increase in the rate of syphilis are the exchange of sexual relations for drugs and decreased resources for syphilis control programs. Individuals with syphilis appear to be at increased risk for HIV infection.

(g) Treatment of syphilis is with penicillin. Primary, secondary, and latent syphilis of less than 1 year's duration are treated with penicillin B benzathine in a single dose. Individuals allergic to penicillin are treated with doxycycline or tetracycline. Pregnant women are treated with penicillin G benzathine. Treatment for syphilis-infected HIV patients is not established.

(2) Nonvenereal syphilis includes three diseases.

(a) Yaws, caused by *T. pertenue,* is a disease that produces lesions of the skin and sometimes bones. It is found in Africa, India, and South America. Treatment is with penicillin.

(b) Pinta is caused by *T. carateum* and also produces lesions. It is found in Central and South America. Treatment is with penicillin.

(c) Bejel is a syphilis primarily of childhood. It is found in the Middle East and is treated with penicillin.

b. The genus *Borrelia,* actively motile spirochetes, are transmitted to human beings by arthropod vectors. The largest of the pathogenic spirochetes are 10 to 30 μm long and 0.3 to 0.7 μm wide. They infect rodents, birds, and domestic animals and cause two diseases in human beings.

   (1) *B. recurrentis* causes relapsing fever transmitted to humans by lice, primarily in Africa. In North America, relapsing fever is caused by *B. hermsii, B. turicatae,* and *B. parkeri,* and is transmitted via ticks that have acquired the microorganisms from rodents. About 15 cases are reported in the United States every year, most often in California, Oregon, Colorado, and Texas. The microorganisms invade the spleen, liver, kidneys, eyes, and brain. An initial attack, presenting with chills, fever, and a rash, lasts three to seven days, and an asymptomatic period ensues. After that, the patient suffers four or more attacks similar to the first but of decreasing severity and duration. Treatment is with tetracyclines and chloramphenicol.

   (2) Lyme disease is transmitted to human beings by ixodid ticks that are infected with *B. burgdorferi.* It is a chronic inflammatory disease, most frequently reported in the United States, and first reported in Lyme, Connecticut, in 1977. There are two stages of the disease.

      (a) In the first stage a lesion at the site of the tick bite, called an erythema chronicum migrans (ECM), develops and the symptoms are headache, low fever, stiff neck, and arthralgia. Red-brown or purple lesions may also appear on the ear lobes, nipples, scrotum, and extremities. This stage lasts from 3 to 14 days.

      (b) The second stage causes arthritis in the large joints, such as the knees, along with intense pain in tendons, bursa, and muscles. This stage occurs weeks or months after the first stage. In about 15% of patients, neurological involvement, including meningoencephalitis and facial palsy, occurs. The people who have been infected are constantly fatigued and experience altered mental states. Effects of the disease may be chronic, lasting years after the original infection.

(c) Treatment of the disease, initially, is through the administration of doxycycline and amoxicillin. Treatment of the later stage is through ceftriaxone or cefotaxime. Recurrent fever is treated with tetracyclines and chloramphenicol. Prevention of the disease is based on attempts to control the vectors through the use of insecticides and people's careful attention to the possible presence of ticks after they have been in areas where the insects are common.

(3) Species of the genus *Leptospira* that are pathogenic to human beings are members of the group *L. interrogans*. These are spiral-shaped organisms, having coils and hooked ends. They are harbored by wild rodents and domestic animals and are shed in animal urine. Infrequent in the United States, infection is the result of contaminated water or soil that contacts abrasions of the skin. The organisms infect the liver, lungs, and meninges. Serious infections cause jaundice and a resultant high mortality rate. Treatment is with penicillin, ampicillin, tetracyclines, and cephalosporins.

2. Spiral and curved rods differ from the spirochetes in that their motility is the result of the presence of polar flagella rather than axial filaments.

   a. The only human pathogen of the genus *Spirillum* is *S. minor,* which causes rat-bite fever. This infection is transmitted to human beings via the bite of an infected cat or rat and causes a rash and an enlargement of the lymph nodes. The disease is usually self-limiting.

   b. Members of the genus *Campylobacter* are the most frequent cause of gastroenteritis in developed countries today. *C. jejuni, C. coli,* and *C. fetus,* are most often the causative agents. They are ingested by human beings in contaminated poultry and meat, though contaminated water is sometimes the source of infection. Direct transmission occurs among butchers and poultry processors. Infections are not always symptomatic, so carriers are a factor in the spread of the disease. When symptoms do occur they include diarrhea, abdominal pain, fever, and myalgia. Guillain-Barré syndrome has been associated with infection by *C. jejune*. Infection is usually self-limiting. Prevention of *campylobacter* infection is accomplished through pasteurization of milk and proper handling of raw poultry and meat.

   c. *Helicobacter pylori* is considered to be the major cause of chronic gastritis. Its presence in the human stomach, causing chronic inflammation of the stomach and duodenum, may predispose people to peptic ulcers. Treatment is with metronidazole or tinidazole, along with amoxicillin or tetracycline and bismuth salt.

K. Mycoplasmas and L-forms
1. Mycoplasmas do not have cell walls, yet are able to survive without invading other organisms. Most are aerobes or facultative anaerobes, but a few species are anaerobic. They are so small (0.2 to 0.3 μm) that they can pass through bacterial filters. They are pleomorphic and assume coccoid, filamentous, or cocci in chains as their forms. Sterols are contained in their cytoplasmic membranes, and these are not found in any other bacterial cells.
   a. *M. pneumoniae* is the cause of atypical or walking pneumonia in children and young adults. Transmission of infection is through aerosolized respiratory secretions and is common in institutions.
   b. *U. urealyticum* and *M. hominis* are opportunistic pathogens that cause genitourinary tract infections in sexually active people. They can be transmitted to infants as they pass through the birth canal. *U. urealyticum* causes nongonococcal urethritis that can cause premature spontaneous labor and delivery, resulting in stillbirths and perinatal deaths from pneumonia, septicemia, and meningitis.
   c. *M. hominis* also causes PID, postpartum fever, pyelonephritis, bacteremia, and wound and joint infections.
   d. *M. genitalium* causes acute nongonococcal urethritis. Treatment of infections by mycoplasmas is with erythromycin and tetracyclines.
2. L-forms are wall-deficient bacteria that may or may not revert to normal cell structure at various times. Development of L-forms are considered to be a survival mechanism for

the cells that are under unusual circumstances such as being in the presence of penicillin. L-forms can only be isolated on media that have a high concentration of nonmetabolizable solute, such as sodium chloride, that creates a high osmotic pressure gradient.

L. Rickettsiae and Chlamydiae

1. Rickettsial species have cell walls similar to gram-negative organisms but are pleomorphic and usually take the shape of rods. They are intracellular parasites, except the genus *Rochalimaea.*

   a. All members of the family Rickettsiae (except *Coxiella burnetii*) are transmitted to human beings via insect vectors. They are harbored in mice and ticks, and human infection occurs when ticks, mites, lice, or fleas are crushed at the site of a bite. Diseases caused by the organisms are classified into five groups.

   (1) The typhus group

      (a) Epidemic or louse-borne typhus is caused by *Rickettsia prowazekii,* which often causes epidemics in Ethiopia, central Africa, and South America. Death comes through myocardial and neurological involvement. People who survive the disease can become carriers of the organism. The disease occurs in the eastern and southeastern United States in a form called sylvatic typhus, which is associated with flying squirrel lice. Sylvatic typhus is a milder form of illness.

      (b) A mild form of typhus transmitted to human beings via rat fleas is endemic or murine typhus, caused by *R. typhi.* It occurs infrequently in the United States.

   (2) The spotted fever group

      (a) Rocky Mountain Spotted Fever is caused by *Rickettsia rickettsii* and is the most frequently reported rickettsial disease in the United States, most often in children and young adults. The American dog tick is responsible for transmitting the disease, originally from rabbits, raccoons, foxes, woodchucks, and deer, to human beings in the eastern United States, primarily in Mississippi, Virginia, North Carolina, and Tennessee. In the western states, the wood tick is responsible for transmission. Symptoms of the disease are fever, headache, lymphadenopathy, and usually, rash. Symptoms are often misdiagnosed as measles, rubella, encephalitis, or meningococcemia. Death can result from progressive hypotension that leads to convulsions, intravascular coagulation, or cardiac arrest, usually within 10 days after the appearance of symptoms. Death often occurs because inappropriate antibiotic therapy is administered based on an incorrect diagnosis.

(b) Mediterranean Spotted Fever (also called boutonneuse fever) is caused by tick-borne *Rickettsia conorii* and is similar to Rocky Mountain Spotted Fever, though seldom fatal.

(c) Siberian tick typhus is caused by *Rickettsia sibirica* and is a mild disease.

(d) Rickettsial pox is caused by *Rickettsia akari* and is found in North America, the former Soviet Union, South Africa, and Korea. Queensland tick typhus is caused by *Rickettsia australis* and is found in Australia.

(3) Scrub typhus is caused by *Rickettsia tsutsugamushi* and occurs in eastern Asia and islands of the South Pacific. If untreated, it causes respiratory, neurological, and cardiovascular complications, but it can be successfully treated with antibiotics.

(4) Q fever was originally given the designation *Q* for the word *query,* which referred to "fever of unknown origin." Most cases are found in Australia and Great Britain, but the disease can occur anywhere in the world. Q fever is caused by *C. burnetii* and is a zoonosis—transmitted to human beings from sheep, goats, cattle, and ticks. Animals place the organism in the human environment in milk, urine, feces, and afterbirth, and the organisms can

survive for long periods. Most often, people acquire the disease via inhalation of aerosolized organisms from dried afterbirth tissue and the fluids of farm animals. The organism is believed to form spores. Inhalation of a single organism can result in disease. Infection causes high fever, headache, cough, myalgia, and chest pain. Pneumonia, hepatitis, and endocarditis can result from infection but are rare. Treatment is with tetracycline.

   (5) Trench fever is caused by *Rochalimaea quintana* and is transmitted from person to person via lice. It was major disease during World War I and World War II but now is a minor disease.

  b. *Ehrlichia* have recently been found to cause diseases in human beings. *E. sennetsu* causes glandular fever in Japan and Malaysia and resembles infectious mononucleosis. *E. canis* and *E. chafeensis* cause a disease, thought to be transmitted via the brown dog tick, that resembles Rocky Mountain Spotted Fever. Severe infections can cause respiratory insufficiency, renal insufficiency, and central nervous system involvement.

  c. *Rochalimaea* cause several diseases in human beings.

   (1) Cat-scratch disease causes chronic lymphadenopathy in children and adults, which begins as a lesion that heals. The species involved are *Rochalimaea henselae* (90%) and *Afipia felis,* which causes the remainder. Usually, the disease resolves itself, but serious infections are treated with erythromycin, doxycycline, and rifampin.

   (2) Bacillary angiomatosis is caused by *R. henselae* and causes infections most often in HIV-infected patients. It is thought to be the same infection that causes cat-scratch disease.

2. The chlamydiae are intracellular parasites with cell walls similar to gram-negative bacteria. Members of the genus *Chlamydia* have a developmental cycle, during which the microorganism exists in two forms: the elementary body, which is the extracellular infectious form, and the reticulate body, which is the intracellular noninfectious form.

a. *Chlamydia trachomatis* is the leading cause of sexually transmitted disease in the United States, and worldwide it is the cause of blindness in 9 million people.
   (1) Nongonococcal urethritis in men is caused by *C. trachomatis* and is asymptomatic in up to one-third of the men infected. The disease is, thus, often untreated, and the organism is transmitted sexually to the cervix of a female sexual partner. In the event that a man is symptomatic, the symptom does not appear for 2 to 3 weeks, and unknowing transmission can occur during that period.
   (2) Infection in women is initially asymptomatic, but PID can eventually develop in 2% to 18% of infected women, and *C. trachomatis* is associated with sterility in those patients. The highest rates of infections in both men and women are in those with multiple sexual partners.
   (3) *C. trachomatis* is the causative agent in lymphogranuloma venereum, a sexually transmitted disease that is relatively rare in the United States.
   (4) Trachoma is a chronic ocular disease caused by repeated infections by *C. trachomatis*. In India, Africa, and parts of the south-central areas of the United States, it is endemic. The organism is spread by contaminated hands, washcloths, clothing, linens, and by direct contact between parents and children. Infection of the conjunctiva eventually causes the upper eyelid to turn in, causing abrasions of the cornea by the eyelashes. Blindness is the result.
      (a) Inclusion conjunctivitis is the result of ocular chlamydial infection that does not cause blindness. Infants are infected as they pass through the birth canal, and the result is called ophthalmia neonatorum. Neonatal pneumonia can also result from infection acquired in this manner.
      (b) Inclusion conjunctivitis in adults is acquired primarily from contact with contaminated water in swimming pools. The disease is usually self-limiting in both infants and adults.

(5) Psittacosis is caused by *C. psittaci* that is harbored primarily in birds and is usually asymptomatic when transmitted to human beings. Transmission is through direct contact and causes chills, fever, and atypical pneumonia.

(6) *C. pneumoniae* is transmitted from person to person, primarily in the elderly, and causes pneumonia. *C. pneumoniae* (once called TWAR, for Taiwan Acute Respiratory) causes about 300 000 cases of pneumonia annually in the United States. While most infections are mild, the recovery period is lengthy. The organism also causes sinusitis in young adults.

(7) Treatment for most chlamydial disease is with doxycycline and azithromycin, though erythromycin, amoxicillin, and cephalosporins are used in certain situations.

M. *Actinomyces*

Members of the genus *Actinomyces* are facultative anaerobes that are part of the microflora of the oral cavity, intestinal tract, and pelvic area. They exhibit characteristics of both bacteria and fungi, in that they have prokaryotic cell walls and the ability to form branches or filament. Many species are used in the commercial production of antibiotics. Disease caused by members of the species is called actinomycosis.

1. The most common type of actinomycosis is cervicofacial-causing infection, usually in the lower jaw, and is associated with tooth decay, jaw fracture, or tooth extraction. Serious untreated infections can invade the orbital cavity, causing blindness.

2. Thoracic infection is the result of aspiration, extension of oral infection, or hematogenous spread. Lesions develop in the lung tissue and spread to the pleura, causing a fever and a cough resembling those of TB.

3. Abdominal actinomycosis is associated with trauma to the abdominal wall and perforated appendices.

4. Genital infection is associated with the use of intrauterine devices (IUDs) and the resulting breakdown of the endometrium.

5. Treatment of actinomycoses includes the surgical debridement of infected tissue and the administration of penicillin G or trimethoprim and sulfamethoxazole.

N. *Nocardia*

Members of the genus *Nocardia* are aerobic organisms found in the soil and water. They cause infections in patients who are undergoing immunosuppressive therapy and in those with chronic pulmonary disease. Infections can involve the nervous system and the kidneys, producing fatalities in up to 80% of cases. Treatment includes surgical debridement and the administration of clotrimazole or sulfadiazine.

O. *Legionella*

The causative agent of Legionnaires' disease is *L. pneumophila,* a gram-negative, aerobic bacillus that is a facultative intracellular parasite. The organism is normally found in fresh water and wet soil.

1. It can also be isolated from water systems in buildings, including pipes and rubber and plastic washers and fittings. Within water systems, *L. pneumophila* are often engulfed by ameba and so are protected from the chlorination of the water. Transmission has been associated with aerosols from cooling towers, heat-exchange apparatus, shower heads, and tap water.

2. There were 1280 cases of Legionnaire's disease in the United States in 1993. Many infections occur in patients who have predisposing factors. Outbreaks are more common in the summer, and it is believed that this is the result of contact with contaminated aerosols from air conditioning systems as well as contact with contaminated recreational water.

3. Infection causes fever, lethargy, disorientation, severe bronchopneumonia with inflammation in the respiratory bronchioles, and alveoli.

4. *L. pneumophila* also causes Pontiac fever, which is a self-limiting, influenzalike illness that is not fatal.

5. Treatment of the disease is with erythromycin. Elimination of the organism from water systems is difficult.

XI. **Viruses**

Viruses are unique obligate intracellular microorganisms that range in size from 20 to 300 nm. Viruses have either DNA or RNA, plus a protein capsid (coat).

A. Viral Classification

Viruses are presently classified according to
- the symptoms of the diseases that they cause

- the method of their transmission
- the symmetry of the virus capsid
- the tissue or organ affected by the virus

B. Entry of the Host
1. Viruses usually enter their mammalian hosts through the respiratory tract and the gastrointestinal tract and the bites of arthropods or through skin abrasions. Transmission may be from one individual to another, which is called horizontal transmission, or from a mother to a fetus, which is called vertical transmission.
2. Entry into the host cell occurs in three ways.
   a. Endocytosis refers to a virus that binds to the surface of a cell membrane.
   b. Fusion occurs when a virus fuses with a cell's cytoplasmic membrane.
   c. Direct penetration occurs when a virus is so small that it is able to pass directly through the cytoplasmic membrane into the cytoplasm.

C. Viral Replication
After entering a host cell, viruses replicate in a number of ways.
1. They attach to the host cell and are absorbed through the surface of the host cell.
2. They penetrate the cell.
3. The virus loses its coating.
4. Viral nucleic acids and proteins biosynthesize.
5. Virions assemble (complete virus particles form).
6. Virus particles release via budding through the membrane of the host cell.

D. Antiviral Agents
Viruses can be inactivated or rendered noninfective by a variety of means.
1. Agents that react with viral protein
   a. Radiation in the form of ultraviolet light at wavelengths of 2350Å destroys proteins.
   b. Temperatures of 55°C to 65°C for 1 hour inactivate most proteins except polio and serum hepatitis viruses.
   c. Proteolytic enzymes can inactivate some viruses.

    d. Phenol also alters viruses so that they are inactive.
2. Agents that react with viral nucleic acids
    a. Formaldehyde reacts with the amino groups of viral nucleic acids but does not render viruses inactive. It is used in the preparation of viral vaccines.
    b. The use of nitrous acid causes mistakes in the replication of viral DNA.
    c. Radiation with ultraviolet light at wavelengths of 2600Å inactivates RNA and DNA viruses.
3. Photodynamic inactivation is a process that involves staining the virus with a dye and then irradiating it with visible light.
E. Chemotherapy

Since most antibacterial drugs act in specific ways to inhibit bacteria, especially against bacterial cell walls, they are not effective against viruses.

1. Antivirals

Agents that are successful against viral infection are nucleoside analogues, but they are toxic to the host (see Appendix C). Immunoglobulins, primarily prophylactically, are used as antiviral agents. Hyperimmune globulins are used for postexposure, prevention of hepatitis B, chickenpox, and rabies.

2. Vaccines

Immunization is extremely important in the prevention of epidemics of viral diseases. Vaccines are of three types.

    a. Live vaccines are prepared from viruses that are still alive but are so attenuated (weakened) that they only stimulate the formation of antibodies but do not produce the symptoms of the disease. They are used to prevent poliomyelitis, rubella, yellow fever, measles, adenovirus, mumps, and chickenpox.

    b. Inactivated vaccines are prepared from viruses that have been treated with formaldehyde, phenol, or betapropiolactone. Vaccines against infection with influenza A, rabies, and poliomyelitis are used.

    c. Recombinant subunit vaccines are developed from genetically altered viruses. The hepatitis B vaccine is an example.

XII. DNA Viral Diseases

A. Poxviruses

The most important genus of this family is *Orthopoxvirus*, which contains the species *variola virus* and *monkeypox virus*. *Variola virus* is the causative agent of smallpox, which caused 49 000 cases and 173 deaths in the United States in 1930–1931, 134 years after the introduction of the vaccine by Edward Jenner. The disease was declared eradicated by the World Health Organization in 1977. Smallpox is transmitted by inhaling the virus from lesions found in the oropharynx of infected people. Small amounts of the virus are stored in Atlanta and Moscow, and there is a debate over whether they should be destroyed. Vaccination for *variola virus* is recommended for some laboratory workers. Monkeypox is a disease of monkeys in Africa and Asia. The virus can be transmitted to human beings, but it is a rare disease.

B. Herpesviruses

Herpeviruses cause several latent infections that in turn cause recurrent infections.

1. Cytomegalovirus (CMV)

Cytomegaloviruses frequently cause infections in infants, renal-transplant patients, those receiving immunosuppressive drugs, and those with acquired immune deficiency syndrome (AIDS).

a. In the United States, congenital CMV disease is the most common serious infection in newborns. Fetuses become infected through the placentas of infected mothers, and the infection affects nearly every organ of the fetus. Of all infants in the United States, 1% have congenital CMV infection. Of those, 90% have subclinical disease that will remain chronic, 5% to 10% will experience symptoms that include retardation of intrauterine growth, hepatosplenomegaly, jaundice, deafness, and chorioretinitis. CMV causes mental retardation in about 5% of infected infants. Infection can also be acquired postpartum from the mother's mouth or milk.

b. More than 90% of renal-transplant patients become infected with CMV either from donated kidneys or from blood transfusions. CMV causes pulmonary and hepatic complications.

c. AIDS patients are also susceptible to CMV infections.

d. Methods through which CMV are transmitted are congenital transfer, direct contact with donor organs, blood transfusions, and contact with infected body fluids. CMV is often transmitted in day-care facilities, and within families, and is spread through sexual contact.

e. Treatment of the infection is with ganciclovir. Acyclovir is given prophylactically to bone-marrow and kidney-transplant recipients.

2. Varicella-zoster virus

a. Chickenpox (varicella) and shingles (zoster) are manifestations of the same disease in different age groups. Chickenpox is normally a self-limiting disease, but superinfections of streptococci or staphylococci can cause complications. In adults, the disease can cause pneumonia. In immunodeficient or immunosuppressed patients, varicella infection can be fatal.

b. Shingles (zoster) results from the reactivation of the varicella virus in posterior root or cranial sensory nerve ganglia. Reactivation is believed to be the result of immunosuppression. Lesions and rash appear, and postherpetic neuralgia that develops later may last up to 6 months, especially in patients over 60. AIDS patients and other immunosuppressed patients often develop zoster.

c. Varicella is a very contagious disease and is believed to be transmitted by the airborne route. One hundred and forty-five cases are reported in the United States each year. Humans are thought to be the only reservoir for the virus. Infection results in permanent immunity in most people.

d. Usually varicella infection produces a self-limiting disease, but studies have shown that the administration of acyclovir decreases the pain caused by the disease and accelerates healing. A vaccine has recently been approved for use in the United States.

3. Herpes simplex virus

There are two serotypes of herpes simplex virus (HSV). Type 1 (HSV-1) causes lesions in the oral cavity and facial areas, and type 2 (HSV-2) causes infection primarily in the genital area. Either type can cause infection at any body site. Infection can be either primary or recurrent. The virus, after infection, remains in the nerve axons and sensory ganglia.

a. Type 1 infections

(1) Acute herpetic gingivostomatitis produces ulcerative lesions in the oral cavity. It is self-limiting.

(2) Eczema herpeticum causes lesions of the skin.

(3) Herpetic keratoconjunctivitis leads to opacity of the cornea and is the leading cause of loss of vision by external causes in the United States.

(4) Herpes labialis causes fever blisters and cold sores. Recurrent reactivation of the virus at these sites is believed to be the result of stress, sunlight, hormones, menstruation, and dental extractions.

(5) Herpetic encephalitis is thought to be acquired through the nasal cavity. Infection occurs soon after birth and often causes death within 3 weeks. Both HSV-1 and HSV-2 are associated with this disease, although HSV-2 creates more brain damage in infants and HSV-1 does so in adults.

b. Type 2 infections

(1) Genital herpes is a disease occurring most often in adolescents and young adults. Infection in children is a sign of sexual abuse. Many infected persons are asymptomatic or have subclinical infection, but the disease can produce lesions on the vagina, cervix, and vulva in female patients and on the penis in male patients. Previous infection with HSV-1 reduces susceptibility to HSV-2 infection. People infected with genital herpes are infected for life and are intermittent shedders of the virus. In the United States, more than 30 million people are infected with genital herpes.

(2) Neonatal herpes is contracted from infected mothers and is more serious when the infection is the mothers' first infection. The disease often results in

• disseminated infection, which produces a mortality rate of 80%.

- Central nervous system infection which produces a mortality rate of 50%. Of the survivors, fewer than 10% will develop normally.
- Skin, eye, or mouth infection, which, untreated, eventually leads to either disseminated disease or infection of the central nervous system in 75% of cases.

(3) Herpetic whitlows are lesions caused by contact with HSV lesions of either type 1 or type 2. They are associated with medical personnel and heal after about 1 month.

(4) Treatment of HSV infections is with acyclovir, vidarabine, or foscarnet. Vidarabine is administered intravenously for herpes encephalitis and neonatal herpes. Trifluridine and idoxuridine in solutions are used to treat herpes keratitis.

4. Epstein-Barr virus (EBV)
   EBV is usually established early in childhood.
   a. Exposure to EBV causes infectious mononucleosis in about two-thirds of adolescents and young adults who are exposed to it. The most important method of transmission is via saliva. The disease causes sore throat, fever, fatigue, enlarged cervical lymph nodes, and splenomegaly. Fifteen to twenty percent of young adults are shedders, as are infected immunosuppressed patients, such as AIDS patients. The disease usually resolves in a month but long-lasting fatigue can occur. Complications of infection include hemolytic anemia, aplastic anemia, and agranulocytosis.
   b. Infection with EBV can also cause a disease that lasts for months or years called chronic mononucleosis syndrome. Chronic mononucleosis produces intermittent or persistent fever, lymphadenopathy or hepatosplenomegaly, and other complications but is rarely life threatening. There is no treatment for this syndrome.
   c. In immunosuppressed patients in general, EBV infections can be life threatening. In AIDS patients, EBV infection causes oral hairy leukoplakia, malignant lymphoma, lymphadenopathy, and lymphoid interstitial pneumonitis.

5. Human herpesvirus-6 (HHV-6)
   HHV-6 is thought to be acquired early in life, thus establishing a latent infection. It has been very strongly linked to chronic fatigue syndrome and is found in AIDS patients who have lymphoma and leukemia.
C. The Adenoviruses
   The adenoviruses can be found in many animals, including human beings. In human beings, they are associated with the mucocutaneous surfaces and produce respiratory illness, especially in infants; ocular diseases; and gastrointestinal illness. Nearly every child in the United States has had at least one adenovirus infection by the time they reach the age of 5 years.
   1. The virus causes respiratory disease, primarily in children under 6 years of age. Five to twenty-five percent of acute respiratory disease in hospitalized children is caused by the virus. As well, it causes pharyngitis, bronchitis, croup, and pneumonia in children in general. Infections have been associated with "swimming pool" conjunctivitis and lower respiratory tract disease, also.
   2. Keratoconjunctivitis outbreaks in industry and in ophthalmologists' offices are caused by adenovirus.
   3. Adenovirus often causes gastroenteritis, especially in infants, on a worldwide basis.
   4. No chemotherapeutic agent is effective in treating adenovirus infection, but a vaccine is available.
D. The Papillomaviruses
   The human papillomaviruses (HPV) are the cause of warts.
   1. There are four types of warts, and each type is treated with specific therapy. The types are verruca vulgaris (common wart), verruca plana (flat wart), verruca plantaris (plantar wart), and condylomata acuminata (venereal warts). Usually, warts regress, but if they do not, they are treated with electrosurgery, cryosurgery, and topical drugs such as podophyllotoxin or trichloroacetic acid.
   2. Venereal warts appear on the external genitalia and the rectum and are very commonly transmitted. Between 12 and 14 million people in the United States are infected with this sexually transmitted disease. In children, the disease is usually acquired during the birth process or via nonsexual hand-genital family contact but may be a sign of sexual

abuse. Almost 30% of women with venereal warts also have gonorrhea, and most homosexual men with perianal warts also have syphilis or gonorrhea.

3. Some papillomavirus infections produce lesions that are not readily visible because the disease is subclinical, but they can still be transmitted to neonates, resulting in laryngeal papillomatosis.

E. The Parvoviruses

Parvovirus B 19 causes erythema infectiosum (fifth disease), a mild, epidemic disease in children. The name *fifth disease* refers to a previously used system in which children's diseases were assigned numbers. The disease is transmitted via respiratory secretions and causes a rash resembling rubella. It is self-limiting in children, but in adults it can cause arthralgia or arthritis, fatigue, and depression. Infection during pregnancy is associated with the risk of spontaneous abortion, stillbirth, or delivery of a hydropic infant. Hydrops fetalis causes severe, aplastic anemia and myocarditis. Pregnant health care workers should not care for patients with B 19 induced aplastic crisis, but neonates infected in utero are not a risk for transmission.

XIII. RNA Viral Diseases

A. Measles Virus

Measles infection is spread to the respiratory tract, mouth, pharynx, and conjunctiva, and during the incubation period of 7 to 10 days causes fever, conjunctivitis, sore throat, headache, and photophobia. A rash then appears. The patient is highly contagious during the incubation period and for up to 2 days after the rash appears.

1. Virus is shed from the conjunctiva and respiratory mucosa. Of those infected, 95% develop characteristic small red macules with bluish-white centers on the inside of the cheeks, called Koplik's spots. Although measles is a self-limiting disease, secondary infections such as pneumonia can occur. Encephalitis occurs in 1 of every 1000 patients, which can result in the loss of mental or motor functions. Rarely does measles infection cause subacute sclerosing panencephalitis, which is fatal.

2. Measles infection during pregnancy can cause premature labor, spontaneous abortions, and low birth-weight infants. Measles infection also causes pneumonitis and hepatitis in pregnant women.

3. Vaccination against measles virus is essential in preventing epidemics of the disease because it is one of the most easily communicable diseases in human beings. The vaccine is available alone or in combinations: measles-rubella (MR) and measles-mumps-rubella (MMR) vaccines.

B. Mumps Virus

The mumps (epidemic parotitis) virus multiplies in the respiratory tract, enters the blood, and infects other organs and the central nervous system. The incubation period is 14 to 21 days. Then, the salivary parotid glands characteristically swell, often painfully. Unilateral infection of the testes occurs in about 25% of infected men.

1. Mumps is usually a benign disease, but complications include pancreatitis, thrombocytopenia, aseptic meningitis, meningoencephalitis (which may or may not cause permanent damage), and orchitis, which if bilateral, may cause sterility.

2. The virus is transmitted via respiratory droplets, or fomites contaminated with saliva. Adding to the contagion risk is the fact that up to 5% of infected persons are asymptomatic, and virus is shed from saliva and urine for several days before symptoms do occur. Today, many outbreaks occur on high schools and college campuses because many young people were not vaccinated and did not have the disease (which results in immunity) at a young age.

3. Mumps vaccine provides long-lasting immunity and may be given in combination, i.e., MMR vaccine. Vaccine is not recommended for pregnant women, immunocompromised patients, or people born before 1957 (who are likely to be naturally immune).

C. Rubella Virus

The disease rubella, also called German measles, causes disease in two ways.

1. Postnatal rubella infection is transmitted via the respiratory tract and spreads to the bloodstream. The incubation period is 14 to 21 days. A rash appears in the nasopharynx and maximal shedding occurs 1 to 2 days before and 3 to 5 days

after the rash appears. Symptoms also include fever, leukopenia, and suboccipital lymphadenopathy. It is a self-limiting disease, but complications of arthritis and arthralgia are common in young women.

2. Congenital rubella syndrome is the result of the infection of the fetus when the mother is infected during pregnancy and is most common when the infection occurs during the first trimester. Infection results in cataracts, glaucoma, pulmonary artery stenosis, meningoencephalitis, and mental retardation. The mortality rate for infants with symptoms at the time of birth is 20%.

3. Rubella infection occurs more frequently during the winter and spring months. It is transmitted via person-to-person contact with both symptomatic and asymptomatic persons able to shed the virus.

4. There is no available treatment for either congenital or postnatal rubella infection. When infection occurs during the first trimester of pregnancy, many physicians recommend therapeutic abortion. Administration of the vaccine results in apparently lifelong protection but can result in a short, subclinical infection. It is not given to women during early pregnancy because fetal infection may occur. Administration of the vaccine can cause arthritis in adults, especially in women.

D. Influenza Viruses

Of the three types of influenza viruses, type A has been found in human beings, horses, swine, and birds, while types B and C have been found only in human beings. Influenza viruses are classified by antigenic type, e.g., A, B, or C; geographical location or origin, e.g., Taiwan; year of isolation, e.g., 1968; strain number, e.g., 5; and antigenic identity of hemagglutinin (H) subtype and neuraminidase (N) subtype. Thus, the name of one particular virus is A/Taiwan/5/68(H2N2).

1. Types A and B viruses cause more severe diseases than do type C viruses. Influenza is acquired via inhalation of aerosols from infected people and infects the upper respiratory tract. After an incubation period of 24 hours, sore throat, fever, cough, headache, muscular aches, and conjunctivitis are experienced for five days. In children, otitis media, croup, and pneumonia may develop. Damage to the mucociliary blanket during infection predisposes patients

to infections by organisms such as *S. aureus, S. pneumoniae,* and *H. influenzae,* and can result in pneumonia, especially in those with underlying disease and in the elderly.

2. A complication of influenza A and B infections (and varicella infection) is Reye's syndrome, which occurs in children between the ages of 6 and 11 years. The disease has been linked to salicylates that have been used to reduce fever during influenza infection. Reye's produces vomiting, lethargy, and delirium. If untreated, the syndrome can be fatal. In addition, some survivors have suffered brain damage. The risk of developing Reye's syndrome is highest following an influenza type B infection followed by varicella-zoster and influenza type A infections.

3. Influenza epidemics occur every 2 to 5 years. Pandemics, which take place every 8 to 10 years, are caused by the influenza A virus. Influenza viruses change through a process known as antigenic drift. This is particularly true of influenza type B viruses, and new influenza subtypes cause pandemics, as occurred in 1957, 1968, and 1977. In 1957, 80 million cases of infection and 88 000 pneumonia-and-influenza related deaths were reported in the United States, mostly among debilitated patients and the elderly. Type C influenza is distributed worldwide and infection occurs primarily in the young, but outbreaks are not usually reported.

4. Influenza infection produces immunity that lasts for 1 or 2 years, but resistance to one strain does not confer resistance to other strains. Treatment both for prophylaxis and therapy for persons at high risk, that is, those with chronic pulmonary, heart, or kidney disease, is with amantadine. Adults are also treated with rimantadine, usually in aerosolized form. Vaccines for type A and B strains provide protection during epidemics and should be administered to the elderly, those with chronic disorders, and residents and staff members of nursing homes. Side effects from vaccination occur most often in children and include fever, allergic response, and Guillain-Barré syndrome in 10 of every million cases. The syndrome is fatal in 5% of those who develop it.

E. Poliovirus
   There were 57 879 cases of paralytic poliomyelitis reported in the United States in 1952. A vaccine was introduced in

1955, and only 9 cases per year were reported during the 1980s. Most cases today are vaccine associated.

1. The virus gains entry to human beings, usually through contaminated food, water, or milk. It infects the tonsils, lymph nodes of the neck, and the small intestine, then enters the bloodstream. During the incubation period, which lasts 10 to 15 days, it is shed in the feces. Infection causes fever, headache, and stiffness of the neck.

   a. In nonparalytic polio, the symptoms subside in a few days and patients recover completely.

   b. In 1% of infected patients, the virus invades the central nervous system and destruction of nerve cells causes atrophy of voluntary muscles. Recovery of muscle function is dependent on the number of available uninjured neurons.

2. There are three poliovirus serotypes, and type 1 causes the most infections in the United States. Poliovirus can infect any age group, but paralytic cases occur most often in adolescents and young adults. Epidemics of poliomyelitis still occur in developing countries. A great irony of the disease is that prior to improvements in sanitation in this century, poliovirus infection was an asymptomatic disease of infants and young children, and infection provided permanent immunity. Also, most women had been infected as infants and passed immunity to their children. As sanitation improved, infants were not exposed to the virus (usually via feces), and so, when exposed as adolescents, contracted a disease that produces paralysis in their age group.

3. Two vaccines against poliovirus in the United States are inactivated poliovirus vaccine (IPV), and oral poliovirus vaccine (OPV).

F. Other Enteroviruses

   Enteroviruses (which include poliovirus and hepatitis A virus) infect human beings in a similar manner as does poliovirus, but other organs are also affected.

1. Echoviruses cause aseptic meningitis, a self-limiting disease that produces the symptoms of headache, fever, vomiting, stiffness of the neck, and muscular weakness. Coxsackie viruses A and B may also cause this disease.

2. Group A Coxsackieviruses cause herpangina, a self-limiting disease affecting primarily children between the ages

of 3 and 10. The symptoms include fever, sore throat, and ulcerated lesions in the oral cavity.

3. Group A and B Coxsackieviruses produce a myocarditis that can affect all age groups, but it is often fatal in neonates. It can result in permanent myocardial damage in other age groups as well.

4. Group B Coxsackieviruses cause pleurodynia, a self-limiting muscular disease in children between the ages of 5 and 15 years and in their parents. The characteristic symptom of the disease is pain in the lower rib cage and upper abdomen.

5. Several Coxsackieviruses and echoviruses cause pharyngitis, which appears in the summer months. It is not the usual viral respiratory infection.

6. Enterovirus 70 and group A Coxsackievirus type 24 cause epidemics of acute hemorrhagic conjunctivitis in tropical areas.

7. Coxsackievirus B and echoviruses cause neonatal disease that can cause cardiac or respiratory distress and death. Infection is usually hospital acquired.

8. Between 10 and 15 million cases of disease are caused by nonpolio enteroviruses in the United States each year, primarily in children younger than 10 years of age. Human beings are the only reservoir for the viruses, which are shed in the stool. The viruses are spread most often during warm weather, through contaminated food, water, and fomites contacted by nasal secretions.

9. There is no antiviral therapy for enteroviral disease (except for poliomyelitis). Proper isolation techniques are essential in preventing the spread of outbreaks in the hospital environment.

G. Rhinoviruses

Infection with rhinoviruses is responsible for 50% of infections that are referred to as common colds. Colds are universal among children under 1, and young adults average 0.7 colds per year.

1. The most frequent symptoms of infection are coryza, sore throat, and cough. Fever is not usually present. The principal method for spreading colds is not thought to be through aerosols generated by sneezing or coughing, but via the hands of infected persons. The organism is spread as the infected person touches fomites or the hands of another

person. Autoinfection via touching the eyes or nose then produces infection.

2. Rhinoviruses differ from enteroviruses in that they are rendered noninfective by environments in which the pH is between 3 and 5. The incubation period for rhinovirus illness is 1 to 3 days, producing coryza (infection causing nasal discharge and watery eyes), sore throat, and cough. In children, infection may cause bronchitis or otitis media. Rhinovirus illnesses occur most often in September and October. Since there is a large number of serotypes of the virus (about 89), the use of vaccines is not practical.

H. Respiratory Syncytial Virus (RSV)

RSV infections are associated with 90 000 hospital admissions and 4500 deaths from lower respiratory tract disease in infants and young children each year in the United States. RSV is the major cause of lower respiratory tract disease in those groups. It is thought that the severity of disease caused by the virus is attributable to the site of infection, which is the bronchioles, thus quickly causing airway obstruction.

1. In normal infants, RSV infection usually causes upper respiratory tract symptoms that resolve without complications.

2. In high-risk infants, such as those with congenital heart disease, prematurity, immunodeficiency, and HIV infection, RSV infection causes lower respiratory tract infections including bronchiolitis, pneumonia, and croup.

3. RSV infections in older children are usually mild.

4. Antibody is passed from mother to fetus, but 2 months after birth, children are especially susceptible to RSV infection.

5. Children hospitalized with RSV infection are a risk for spread of the virus via respiratory secretions to other patients and staff alike, and so must be separated from other patients. Strict hand washing procedures for staff must be followed.

6. Therapy for RSV lower respiratory tract infections includes oxygen, ventilatory support, replacement of fluids, and the administration of aerosolized ribavirin in severe cases.

I. Parainfluenza Viruses

Infections with parainfluenza viruses types 1, 2, and 3 cause respiratory infections in infants and children.

1. Primary infections with types 1, 2, and 3 viruses cause coryza, pharyngitis, bronchitis alone or in combination, and a temperature over 100°F for about 3 days.

2. Infections by types 1 and 2 can extend to the larynx and trachea, causing croup, and can lead to fatal pneumonia.
3. Type 3 virus infection causes bronchopneumonia or bronchitis, usually in the first 3 years of childhood.
4. Therapy for parainfluenza virus infection is supportive care.

J. Rabies Virus

Rabies is an infectious viral disease affecting the central nervous systems of warm-blooded animals, including human beings. Virus found in nature is called street virus, while attenuated virus is called fixed virus.

1. Rabies infection in human beings usually is the result of an infected animal bite, though infection can be via aerosols generated by infected bats and by infected corneal grafts.
2. One characteristic of rabies infection is that the incubation period for human beings ranges from 2 to 16 weeks to several years, depending on the site of infection and the time required for the virus to reach the spinal cord or brain. Infection that is not treated before the eighth day is fatal.
3. Sixty percent of patients experience pain at the site of the bite, and 40% of patients experience itching at the site or in the entire affected limb. Other symptoms can include fever, changes in temperament, and coryza. Patients may become either agitated or paralytic as symptoms develop.
4. Hydrophobia (fear of water) is a classic symptom of rabies and is exhibited as violent, jerky contraction of the diaphragm and accessory muscles of respiration that are triggered by attempts to swallow liquids. Patients also experience feelings of terror, excitement, and generalized convulsions. In fatal cases, the patient first becomes comatose.
5. Between 1980 and 1992, only 16 cases of human rabies were reported in the United States, but the disease is much more common in tropical areas, such as Latin America.
6. The rabies virus' permanent hosts are the skunk, raccoon, weasel, and mongoose, and these animals are the source of infection for dogs, cats, cattle, and horses. In Alaska, the arctic fox transmits rabies, and rabid bats have been identified in all 48 contiguous states. In areas where domestic animals have been vaccinated, human infection results most often from the bites of wild animals.

7. Treatment after a bite from an infected animal, or one that is suspected of being infected, includes flushing the wound with soap and water, application of 40% to 70% alcohol, tincture of iodine, or 0.1% quaternary ammonium compounds, and the administration of human rabies immune globulin (HRIG). This is followed by five doses of human diploid cell virus (HDCV). Preexposure or prophylactic vaccination is with HDCV. Rabies vaccine adsorbed (RVA) is available only in Michigan. Prevention of human rabies should be through vaccination of domestic animals. Various methods are being experimented with in attempts to control the virus in wild animals.

K. Hemorrhagic Fever Viruses

Hemorrhagic fevers, with the exception of dengue viruses, can all be life-threatening diseases. Transmission to human beings is vector borne by ticks and mosquitos, or via the aerosolized excreta of infected rodents. Person-to-person transmission is possible, however. Ten of the 12 hemorrhagic fevers are not usually seen in the United States, but yellow fever and dengue are seen and are described under Arboviruses (see XII L).

1. Lassa fever

The Lassa virus was first identified in Nigeria, and today is the most frequently imported viral hemorrhagic fever in the United States and Europe.

a. The natural host of the virus is the African rat, which excretes contaminated urine near human habitation in rural areas. Infection of human beings occurs through contact with that environment or with contaminated blood. Once infected, people are very contagious and epidemics result.

b. The incubation period is 1 to 3 weeks, and initial symptoms are fever, sore throat, weakness, nonproductive cough, vomiting, and diarrhea. Milder cases then resolve.

c. In severe disease, edema of the face and neck, conjunctival hemorrhage, cyanosis, encephalopathy, and shock develop along with platelet dysfunction. The mortality rate for hospitalized patients is 15% to 20%.

d. Treatment is with ribavirin, which can also help prevent infection if given to people who have had contact with infected patients.

2. Ebola hemorrhagic fever

The Ebola virus, named after a river in Zaire, is transmitted from person to person, but neither the reservoir nor the method of acquiring the infection are known. In 1989, an Ebolalike virus was spread in the United States from macaque monkeys imported from the Philippines. The incubation period is from 2 to 21 days, and symptoms are influenzalike, including fever, myalgia, joint pain, and sore throat followed by diarrhea, abdominal pain, and a rash. Hemorrhaging from the gastrointestinal tract and other sites occurs beginning about the third day of infection. Treatment is supportive because no drug has been effective, and no vaccine is available.

3. Marburg hemorrhagic fever

This disease, named after a town in Germany where research on the virus was done, caused an outbreak when infected material from African green monkeys came into contact with human beings. The incubation period is 3 to 10 days. Secondary transmission of the disease is known to occur from close person-to-person contact, or contact with blood or excretions, and sexual transmission is possible. The reservoir of the virus is not known, nor is the mechanism for its natural acquisition. Treatment is supportive because there is no effective drug and no vaccine available.

4. Crimean-Congo hemorrhagic fever (CCHF)

CCHF is harbored in cattle, sheep, goats, and hares. Ixodid (hard shell) ticks are both reservoirs and vectors for the virus. The disease is endemic in Europe, especially in the former Soviet Union, and has been found in Africa, India, China, and in areas surrounding the Mediterranean Sea. Human infection occurs as the result of a bite by an infected tick; by crushing the tick at the wound site; and by contact with blood, secretions, or excretions of infected animals or human beings. The incubation period is 2 to 9 days. Infection produces symptoms that include fever, headache, myalgia, arthralgia, abdominal pain, vomiting, and a rash. Bleeding and hemorrhaging at multiple sites follows. While some cases are mild, fatality rates can be from 15% to 70%. Treatment is supportive because no drug is effective.

5. Other hemorrhagic fever viruses
   a. The family Arenaviridae causes Argentine HF and Bolivian HF fever.
   b. The family Bunyaviridae causes Rift Valley fever.
   c. The family Flaviviridae causes Kyasanur Forest disease and Omsk hemorrhagic fever.
6. Hemorrhagic fever with renal syndrome (HFRS)
   Four members of the genus *Hantavirus* cause HFRS, found in East Asia, Europe, and on Native-American reservations in the United States. The viruses are harbored in rodents, and infection in human beings causes symptoms of fever, hemorrhage, and renal failure. The viruses cause Adult Respiratory Distress Syndrome in the United States. Treatment is supportive because no antimicrobial agent has proved effective.

L. The Arboviruses
   Members of this group cause several serious arthropod-borne diseases.
   1. Viral encephalitis
      Encephalitis that is caused by members of the arbovirus group is epidemic in nature and includes western equine encephalitis (WEE) virus, eastern equine encephalitis (EEE) virus, St. Louis encephalitis (SEE) virus, and Japanese B encephalitis (JBE) virus. A mild form of the disease is caused by La Crosse virus and is endemic in the eastern United States. Human viral encephalitis is transmitted via mosquitos. EEE virus infections can cause a 30% mortality rate; JBE viral infections in the elderly can result in an 80% mortality rate. The recovery from infection is often prolonged, with symptoms that include sleeplessness, depression, memory loss, and headaches. Some patients suffer speech and gait disturbances. Treatment is supportive because there is no effective drug available.
   2. Yellow fever
      a. Yellow fever is a hemorrhagic fever transmitted to human beings via the bite of a mosquito. Progress of the disease is divided into three periods.
         (1) After a 3- to 6-day incubation period, the patient experiences fever, headache, lumbosacral pain, nausea, and vomiting for about 3 days while the virus is in the bloodstream.

(2) A 1-day period of remission can then occur.

(3) As the virus infects the liver, spleen, kidneys, and heart, the symptoms of jaundice, albuminuria, hemorrhagic manifestations, stupor, delirium, convulsions, and coma develop. The fatality rate is about 20%, with death occurring between 7 and 10 days after infection.

b. Yellow fever develops through two cycles.

(1) Urban fever involves human beings and the *Aedes aegypti* mosquito. This cycle for yellow fever has not been reported in the United States for 30 years as a result of mosquito-control measures.

(2) Jungle or sylvatic yellow fever occurs when infected monkeys are bitten by mosquitos of the genus *Haemogogus,* and the virus is then transmitted to other monkeys or human beings by the mosquito.

c. Treatment is basically supportive, including the administration of intravenous fluids. The vaccine 17 D provides protection against the virus for at least 10 years.

3. Dengue fever and dengue hemorrhagic fever

a. In classic dengue fever, an incubation period of 2 to 7 days follows the bite of an infected *A. aegypti* mosquito after which high fever, headache, lumbosacral pain, myalgia, nausea, and vomiting develop. A rash may appear on the hands, legs, and feet.

b. Although the disease is usually self-limiting, complications can develop, especially in the case of serial infections, and can include hemorrhages, and damage to the liver, vascular system, and reticuloendothelial system. Dengue shock syndrome can result and, if untreated, can produce fatality rates up to 50%.

c. The disease is spread by *A. aegypti* mosquitos in tropical areas, by *Aedes albopictus* in Asia and the Pacific, and now in the United States as a result of used tires containing eggs of the mosquito being imported from Asia.

d. Treatment of classic dengue fever is supportive. For dengue hemorrhagic fever and dengue shock syndrome, plasma replacement, oxygen therapy, and blood transfusions are necessary.

M. Rotaviruses

Rotavirus infection produces acute gastroenteritis in children, primarily in those who live in developing countries. There are three serotypes of rotavirus, but type A causes endemic severe diarrhea in infants and children worldwide.

1. Approximately 110 000 children are hospitalized with rotavirus infections in the United States each year. The virus is transmitted via the fecal-oral route, usually from an older sibling or an adult with subclinical disease and is often spread to day-care centers. The virus can also cause gastroenteritis in adults, and infections in nursing homes can reach the level of 50% of patients.

2. After an incubation period of 48 hours, fever, vomiting, and diarrhea develop, and in children severe lactose intolerance also develops and lasts from 10 to 14 days. Severe infections in children can result in food intolerance, malnutrition, and dehydration, which can be devastating.

3. Infection in neonates produces a mild or asymptomatic disease that results in immunity against severe rotavirus-produced disease but not against symptomatic infection.

4. Treatment consists of replacing fluids and electrolytes. No vaccine is available.

N. Caliciviruses

Infection by caliciviruses causes gastroenteritis in infants, young children, and the elderly, producing symptoms of diarrhea and vomiting. Treatment is the replacement of fluids and electrolytes. No vaccine is available.

O. Norwalk Virus and Astroviruses

1. Norwalk or Norwalklike viruses produce 42% of food-related outbreaks of mild, epidemic gastroenteritis, transmitted via water and shellfish. It produces vomiting, nausea, diarrhea, and abdominal pain. It is a self-limiting disease. Treatment is the administration of fluids. Infection may produce a short-term resistance to further infection.

2. Astroviruses cause gastroenteritis in infants following an incubation period of 24 to 36 hours. Treatment is the administration of fluids and electrolytes.

P. HIV and AIDS

HIV belongs to the retrovirus class named human T lymphotrophic viruses (HTLV). The strain that causes diseases in all areas of the world except West Africa is the HIV-1 strain. In West Africa, the virus that causes infection is HIV-2, which seems to be less virulent than HIV-1. Infection with HIV-1 produces three stages of disease following an incubation period (the time before virus antibodies can be detected) of 6 weeks to 1 year.

1. The primary or acute stage produces symptoms of fever, headache, lymphadenopathy, pharyngitis, myalgias, rash, and infection of CD4+ lymphocytes. About 1 month after their appearance symptoms subside.

2. The chronic or asymptomatic stage follows and lasts from 7 to 11 years, during which time the patient's cell-mediated immune responses deteriorate. The virus changes, replicating much more rapidly than in the first stage and becomes much more destructive to CD4+ cells. Symptoms at this stage that are predictive of the patient's developing AIDS include oral candidiasis, hairy leukoplakia, fever, and weight loss.

3. The crisis or AIDS stage develops when the CD4+ lymphocyte count becomes too low.

   a. This subjects the patient to opportunistic infections including candidiasis of the trachea, bronchi, lung tissue and esophagus; cryptococcosis; cryptosporidiosis; cytomegalovirus disease; Kaposi's sarcoma; *M. avium* and *M. kansasii* infection; *M. tuberculosis* infection (pulmonary or extrapulmonary); *Pneumocystis carinii* pneumonia; herpes simplex infection; histoplasmosis; and other infections.

   b. Disease manifestations at this point include bacillary angiomatosis, thrush (candidiasis), cervical dysplasia and cancer, fever, diarrhea lasting for more than 1 month, hairy leukoplakia, herpes zoster, pelvic inflammatory disease, peripheral neuropathy, and idiopathic thrombocytopenic purpura. Many patients experience AIDS dementia complex, which includes the loss of control over thought and motion in the terminal stage of the disease.

4. Children can acquire AIDS through either horizontal or vertical transmission.

a. Horizontal infection occurs via contact with contaminated blood or blood products, illegal drug injections, and sexual intercourse, including sexual abuse.

b. Vertical transmission occurs via the placenta, during delivery, or through breast-feeding, though the rate of transmission through breast-feeding is low. Vertical transmission is becoming more common because although the percentage of women with AIDS is 10% in the United States, it is about 50% worldwide, and 80% of women who have AIDS are of childbearing age. Transmission from mothers may or may not occur in any particular pregnancy.

c. Children develop symptoms of HIV-1 infection in about 9 months, with 90% of infections being diagnosed by the age of 3. Children rarely develop some of the infections normally seen in adults, but they do develop lymphocytic interstitial pneumonitis much more commonly than do adults. In 50% to 90% of children with AIDS, encephalopathy develops, as do lymphadenopathy, splenomegaly, and hepatomegaly. Those who develop *P. carinii* pneumonia or encephalopathy have a poor prognosis. Most fatalities in HIV-1 infected children occur during the first year of life.

5. Between 1981 and 1992, reported AIDS cases reached 253 488 in the United States. Most of these were in the metropolitan areas of the East and West. Infection is predominantly in homosexual and bisexual men and in injection drug users and their partners. Heterosexual transmission is increasing. More than 17 million people worldwide are infected with HIV.

6. Risk factors for sexual transmission of HIV include the practice of anal intercourse, lack of condom use, and the clinical status of sexual partners. Those people with genital ulcers and uncircumcised men are at increased risk. Those who inject drugs are at risk from shared needles and sexual intercourse with multiple partners.

7. Neither contact of health care workers' skin or mucous membranes with the saliva of HIV-infected people nor daily (nonsexual) contact with infected people has resulted in infection.

8. Treatment of AIDS is through the administration of appropriate chemotherapeutic agents relative to the many opportunistic infections that are encountered as well as the administration of azidothymidine (AZT) or zidovudine, plus dideoxyinosine (DDI), to prevent the transcription of retroviral RNA and DNA. Treatment of *P. carinii* pneumonia often includes aerosolized pentamidine.

9. Precautions against HIV-1 infection include the avoidance of sexual contact with anyone suspected of having AIDS or a positive HIV antibody test, anal intercourse, multiple sexual partners, sexual contact with people who inject illegal drugs, oral-genital contact, and in the past 10 years open-mouth kissing. Men who have had sex with other men should not donate blood, organs, or other tissues. Condoms should be used during sexual intercourse.

Q. Hepatitis Viruses (Table 3–1)

Viral hepatitis is a disease of the liver. Sporadic hepatitis can be caused by several viruses including the CMV and yellow-fever virus, but acute hepatitis is caused by hepatitis A virus (HAV), hepatitis B virus (HBV), hepatitis C virus (HCV), and hepatitis E virus (HEV). Hepatitis referred to as hepatitis D (HDV) is an infection caused by HBV plus HDV.

1. Hepatitis A is usually transmitted via the fecal-oral route through contaminated food, water, milk, and shellfish from contaminated water. Transmission occurs via infected persons who handle food. Outbreaks have been associated with foods such as potato salad, doughnuts, and frozen custards. HAV can also be spread via contaminated blood and blood products, though this is not the usual means of transmission. Hepatitis A infection occurs most frequently in children and adolescents.

a. In the United States, outbreaks of HAV are often associated with day-care centers, especially when the centers accept children younger than 2 years who are not toilet trained or when large numbers of children are enrolled. In the United States 24 238 cases were reported in 1993.

b. The incubation period for hepatitis A is 15 to 50 days, followed by symptoms of fever, headache, and vomiting. Jaundice is not usually present. The disease does not usually cause complications and infection confers

Table 3-1 Epidemiological and Clinical Features of Hepatitis Virus Infection

Characteristic	Hepatitis A	Hepatitis B	Hepatitis C	Hepatitis D	Hepatitis E
Transmission	Fecal–oral route (close personal contact; water and food as vehicles)	Parenteral (IV drug users); sexual contact (homosexual men primarily)	Parenteral (90 percent of posttransfusion-associated cases); IV drug use	Same as for hepatitis B (virus requires presence of hepatitis B virus)	Fecal–oral route
Incubation period	15–50 days	30–150 days	50–70 days	Same as for hepatitis B	10–40 days
Immunity to reinfection	Solid immunity to homologous agent but not heterologous agents	Reinfection with homologous agent possible but seldom occurs; no immunity to heterologous agents	Reinfection believed to occur	Reinfection shown to be possible in animals	Reinfection possible
Complications	Usually none	10% or more become chronic and can lead to liver cancer	Chronic disease may develop	Chronic disease is possible	Chronic disease may develop
Mortality	Less than 1%	1%	Similar to hepatitis B virus	Similar to hepatitis B virus	1–2% in epidemic; 10–20% in pregnant women

Source: Reprinted with permission from *Basic Medical Microbiology,* R.F. Boyd, © 1995, published by Little, Brown & Company.

immunity. There is no treatment for acute hepatitis A infection. Prevention is based on proper sanitation and handwashing after contact with infected persons or contaminated objects. Food workers should be screened for infection before employment.

   c. Human immunoglobulin (IG) is administered to prevent the spread of infection in institutions, among persons in high-risk occupations, and to people who travel to areas of endemic infection. IG prevents infection if given before exposure or less than 2 weeks after exposure and helps prevent epidemic spread.

2. Hepatitis B, in general, is far less infective than is HAV. Transmission is associated with injection drug abuse, heterosexual activity, and homosexual activity. In addition, health care professionals, laboratory workers, oral surgeons, and dentists are at high risk for infection. HBV infection can be either acute or chronic. Infection can range in severity from an asymptomatic infection that completely resolves, to a severe symptomatic infection that can produce 10% mortality.

   a. Hepatitis from HBV infection begins with an incubation period of 30 to 150 days. Symptoms then develop and typically include anorexia, malaise, nausea and vomiting, and often fever. After 3 to 10 days dark urine appears, followed by jaundice lasting 3 to 6 weeks. There is no treatment for acute HBV hepatitis other than liver transplantation in the most serious cases.

   b. Chronic hepatitis may be of two types.

      (1) Chronic persistent hepatitis causes little liver damage and does not cause complications.

      (2) Chronic active hepatitis causes chronic inflammation and necrosis of liver cells, and in 50% of cases progresses to cirrhosis.

   c. HBV infection is associated with liver cancer in western Europe, the United States, and especially in Asia and Africa. The latent period for cancer that is related to HBV is about 30 years.

   d. Transmission of HBV can occur in several ways.

      (1) Mother-to-infant transmission can occur transplacentally, by the oral route at delivery from maternal

blood or stool, or by mother-infant contact immediately after birth. About 3500 infants become chronic carriers each year, and 25% of those die from cirrhosis of the liver or liver cancer.

(2) Transmission can occur through sexual contact. Forty percent of carriers' spouses are infected, and 51% to 76% of homosexual men are infected, as well as 55% to 67% of injection drug users (who tend also to have multiple sexual partners).

(3) Transmission of the virus via the bite of infected mosquitos is possible, but this occurs more often in tropical areas than in the United States.

e. In the United States, it is estimated that 300 000 people become infected with HBV, 4000 die from hepatitis-related cirrhosis, and 800 die from hepatitis-related cancer each year.

f. The Centers for Disease Control estimates that 12 000 health care workers will be infected with HBV each year. Of these, it is estimated that 250 will die from cirrhosis of the liver or liver cancer, and 1200 will become carriers of the virus.

g. The infectiveness of HBV is one of the reasons that universal precautions were developed by the Centers for Disease Control.

h. Blood, blood products, and blood donors must be screened for hepatitis B antigen to prevent the spread of the infection.

i. Hepatitis B vaccine is recommended under preexposure conditions for health care workers with blood or needle-stick exposure, clients and staff of institutions for the developmentally disabled, hemodialysis patients (though not with recombinant vaccine), homosexually active men, injection drug abusers, recipients of some blood products, household members and sexual partners of HBV carriers, and people in some high-risk occupations. Vaccination should be considered for inmates of long-term correctional facilities, heterosexuals with multiple sexual partners, and travelers to high-HBV risk areas.

j. Postexposure vaccine is recommended for infants born to HBV-positive mothers and health care workers having needle-stick exposures to human blood. For those with needle-stick exposures, administration of hepatitis B immune globulin (H BIG) is also recommended.

3. Hepatitis C virus is responsible for nearly 95% of transfusion-related cases of hepatitis as well as most sporadic or community-acquired non-A, non-B hepatitis not associated with transfusion. The major risk factor for the transmission of HCV is injection drug use. Needle sticks, especially from multiply transfused patients, e.g., hemophiliacs and leukemia patients, also are a source of infection as is the practice of tattooing. Sexual transmission and nonsexual household transmission may occur. Treatment for chronic HCV infection is the administration of interferon. Blood and blood products must be tested for HCV.

4. Hepatitis D is transmitted in the same manner as HBV, i.e., sexually, via contaminated needles, and via contaminated blood and blood products. HDV can replicate only in the presence of HBV, and concurrent infection produces a variety of infectious scenarios in different parts of the world that can result in severe liver damage or liver cancer. The administration of interferon is sometimes an effective treatment.

5. Hepatitis E is transmitted by the fecal-oral route and, although not endemic to the United States, HEV causes outbreaks of infection in Asia and Africa, especially in refugee camps. Infection is via contaminated water. It produces symptoms of abdominal pain, arthralgia, and fever. Most patients recover from infection, but in pregnant women the fatality rate is 20%.

R. Slow Virus Infections

Infections with a long incubation period are called slow virus infections and include those commonly seen viruses such as measles virus and polyoma virus or unconventional viral agents called prions. The term *prion* means "proteinaceous infectious particle." Prions are proteins, not viruses or bacteria and are very difficult to identify.

1. Kuru is a degenerative disease, caused by prions and discovered in New Guinea. It is transmitted during the practice of ritualized cannibalism. The infectious agent enters individuals' bodies through skin abrasions, nasal mucosa,

or conjunctiva via the contaminated hands of persons handling infected brain tissue. The latent period for the disease is as long as 2 years, and death occurs 3 to 9 months after the symptoms of tremors and stammering appear. Kuru has virtually disappeared as the practice of cannibalism has been abandoned in New Guinea.

2. Creutzfeldt-Jakob disease, also caused by prions, is a degenerative disease of the central nervous system that affects people between the ages of 35 and 65 and is seen worldwide. Human-to-human transmission occurs via transplantation of corneas and dura matter. The symptoms of the disease include uncoordinated movements and dementia. Death occurs within 9 to 18 months after symptoms appear. There is no treatment for the disease. The virus can be transmitted to primates.

3. Subacute sclerosing panencephalitis (SSPE) is an infection of the nervous system caused by the measles virus (not a prion), occurring most often in children who have had measles before the age of 2. The latent period after measles infections is about 7 years, whereupon the virus appears in the cerebrospinal fluid. Infection produces cerebral changes, convulsive motor signs, coma and spasms, loss of cerebrocortical function, and after 18 months, death. Treatment is with inosine pranobex, which produces long-term remission. The disease is found today primarily in developing countries.

XIV. Fungi

Fungi are eukaryotes, found in the soil as saprophytes, that cause the degradation of organic matter. They range in size and complexity from mushrooms (macroforms), to single-cell yeasts (microforms). Most serious fungal infections in human beings occur in immunocompromised individuals, especially in hospitalized patients. Also, fungal infections are occupational hazards for veterinarians, miners, and nursery personnel. In nature, fungi are very important in the recycling of carbon and other elements as well as in the disposal of chemical wastes. They also, however, destroy many grains, fabrics, and fruits and cause disease in domestic animals. In industry, they are used in the preparation of many products including riboflavin, wine, beer, baker's yeast, soy

sauce, cheese, ethanol, and the pharmaceutical groups, penicillins and cephalosporins.
A. Fungi Forms
    The fungi are divided into two forms.
    1. Yeasts are round or oval single cells, ranging in size from about 4 μm to 24 μm.
    2. Molds are multicellular and are composed of filamentous or tubular structures called hyphae, which may be 5 to 50 μm long and 2 to 4 μm in diameter. They are often partitioned by walls called septa that form compartments that contain cytoplasm and at least one nucleus. In the absence of septa, the cytoplasm and nuclei circulate freely.
        a. As hyphae grow, they intertwine and form a mass called a mycelium, which is divided into a vegetative portion and a reproductive portion.
        b. Some fungi are dimorphic, which means that they can exist as either yeasts or molds.
        c. Fungal cell walls are relatively rigid and thick, compared to bacterial walls, and do not possess a peptidoglycan layer. Major constituents of fungal cell walls are chitin or cellulose that enables them to resist the action of penicillins and cephalosporins.
        d. The cytoplasmic membranes of fungi contain sterols that can be adversely affected by antimicrobials.
        e. Fungi possess an endoplasmic reticulum and organelles, including mitochondria, and a membrane system.
        f. Fungi, except for some aquatic sex cells, do not possess structures of locomotion nor do they, except cryptococcus neoformans, produce capsules.
B. Fungi Classifications
    Fungi are classified in the kingdom Fungi, which makes them distinct from the animal and plant kingdoms. The kingdom Fungi is divided into the Myxomycota or slime molds and the Eumycota, which are pathogenic to human beings. The Eumycota are further divided into
    • zygomycotina, which are opportunistic pathogens
    • ascomycotina, which cause skin infections (dermatophytes) or are pathogenic yeasts
    • basidiomycotina, which include mushrooms
    • deuteromycotina (fungi imperfecti), many of which are pathogenic to human beings

C. Fungal Reproduction
   Fungi reproduce sexually and asexually, but asexual reproduction is more important.
   1. Sexual reproduction involves the union of two nuclei sex cells or sex organs.
   2. Asexual reproduction involves several mechanisms, including
      • fragmentation of a hyphal filament to produce new organisms
      • fission, producing two daughter cells
      • budding, the most common process, producing one new organism from each bud
      • spore formation, with each spore germinating into hyphae that later develop into mycelium. Sporulation occurs in both yeasts and molds and may be brought about by either sexual or asexual means, but asexual sporulation is more important and occurs more frequently than does sexual sporulation.
      a. Sexual sporulation rarely occurs in infected human beings. The sexual phase of fungi is referred to as the perfect state. Sexual spores are of four types.
         (1) Oospores result from the fertilization of female structures.
         (2) Zygospores result from the union of two hyphae.
         (3) Ascospores are found in a sac called an ascus.
         (4) Basidiospores are formed by mushrooms, puffballs, and other large fungi.
      b. Fungi that form spores only asexually are referred to as being in the imperfect state. Asexual spores are produced in either specialized structures or from modified hyphae and are called conidia. They vary in size, shape, and color. Asexual spores that are produced within a specialized sac are called sporangium. Asexual spores arising directly from hyphae are called thallospores, and they are further classified as arthrospores, chlamydospores, and blastospores.
D. Other Characteristics of Fungi
   1. All molds are aerobic, but yeasts are facultative anaerobes.
   2. Fungi can grow on many substrates and can tolerate pHs between 2.0 and 9.0, growing most rapidly at pHs between 5.0 and 6.0.

3. Fungi are cultivated on special low-pH media called Sabouraud agar to prevent the growth of contaminating bacteria on the culture.

E. Pathogenesis

Most fungal species that cause disease in human beings are soil saprophytes, except the *Candida* species. Fungi release thousands of environmentally resistant spores that are disseminated by air or water. Even though fungal spores are commonly ingested or inhaled by human beings, they rarely cause disease unless they are present on objects that penetrate the skin. Most fungal infections in human beings are the result of occupational hazards or constant contact with the soil, or they occur in those with depressed immune systems.

1. Fungal diseases are referred to as mycoses and occur in healthy human beings only if the number of spores is great and they make contact with tissue that can support their growth.

2. Most fungi that infect human beings are opportunistic pathogens.

3. Dimorphic fungi, such as *Histoplasma, Coccidioides, Blastomyces, Sporothrix,* and *Paracoccidioides* can change their form to enable them to grow at 37°C in living tissue.

4. Fungal diseases are classified according to the tissue that they infect. The types are
   • subcutaneous
   • cutaneous
   • superficial
   • opportunistic

F. Diagnosis of Fungal Disease

Diagnosis of fungal disease is made by direct microscopic observation, culture technique, and serological testing. Laboratory procedures that are used include Gram stain, periodic acid-Schiff stain, and Wright stain.

G. Barriers to Fungal Infection

The principal barriers to fungal infection of the human body are the skin and mucous membranes. Inhaled spores are filtered by the respiratory system on the basis of size and density. Antibodies, complement, and cell-mediated immunity provide defenses when the physical barriers are broached, e.g., by burns, wounds, or invasive medical devices.

H. Treatment
Fungal infections are difficult to treat because of the similarity of fungal membranes and organelles to those of human cells. Therefore, drugs that are toxic to fungal cells are toxic to their hosts. Further, there are no vaccines available to prevent fungal disease.

XV. **Fungal Diseases**
Fungal diseases can be classified according to the type of tissue that they infect.
A. Systemic Diseases
Human beings acquire systemic mycoses by inhaling spores of dimorphic fungi found in the soil. Infection begins with pulmonary infection that may or may not be symptomatic and that progresses to other organs.
1. Histoplasmosis is the most common respiratory mycotic infection in human beings. It is caused by *Histoplasma capsulatum* and is found worldwide. In the United States, infection is found most frequently in the Mississippi Valley. Although millions of people are infected, less than 5% are symptomatic.
   a. *H. capsulatum* is found in nitrogen-enriched soil, especially if the soil contains avian fecal material. It is found in chicken houses, starling roosts, and bat caves. Infection is via inhalation of conidia in aerosolized avian excretions. There is no human-to-human transmission.
   b. *H. capsulatum* is an intracellular parasite that attacks the reticuloendothelial system. In acute asymptomatic disease, the lung lesion may calcify and heal, resembling tuberculosis. Disseminated histoplasmosis occurs frequently in leukemic patients in areas where it is endemic. The symptoms of infection are fever and liver, spleen, and lymph node enlargement. In endemic areas, histoplasmosis is a common opportunistic infection in AIDS patients and causes pneumonia that is similar to *P. carinii*.
   c. Treatment is with amphotericin B, itraconazole, or fluconazole.
2. Coccidioidomycosis
This disease is caused by *Coccidioides immitis* and begins as an upper respiratory tract infection that in healthy indi-

viduals is self-limiting. In immunocompromised patients, it can become a disseminated disease that results in fatality.

a. Coccidioidomycosis is found only in the Western hemisphere and in the United States, primarily in the lower Sonoran Desert life zone. Arthroconidia released from the mycelium, which is found in the soil, are carried by the wind and inhaled by human beings.

b. Although the disease occurs in all age groups and races, infection is more serious in children and the elderly. Disseminated disease occurs more commonly in Filipinos, African-Americans, Hispanics, and Native Americans.

c. Epidemics are associated with construction projects, archeological digs, and exploration for oil in sandy soil. Infection can be life threatening in AIDS patients.

d. Of infected persons, 60% are asymptomatic, but the symptoms, when they occur, include mild fever, headache, myalgia, and fatigue. In 5% of symptomatic patients the symptoms are more severe and include plural pain. Disseminated disease develops in only 1% of infected persons, but in those who do develop it, nearly every organ is affected, including the skin and bones. Coccidioidomycosis may develop into meningitis, which can cause death within a few weeks.

e. Treatment for mild infections is the administration of ketoconazole and fluconazole. For severe disease, amphotericin B is recommended.

3. Blastomycosis
Human beings acquire blastomycosis by inhaling spores of the fungus *Blastomyces dermatitidis.* The disease can be chronic and produces granulomatis lesions that may lead to disseminated disease.

a. The disease is endemic in the southeastern United States (except in Florida) in areas with high acidic pH, high organic content, and high moisture. Outbreaks have been associated with cabin construction, work near beaver structures, and excavation sites.

b. Infection produces an acute pulmonary phase that may be asymptomatic, self-limiting, or may produce fulminant infection that may become progressive. Symptoms of infection are cough and fever of 3 days or longer, plural pain, night sweats, and weight loss. Although pulmonary lesions may heal, chronic cutaneous disease can develop, producing lesions on the face, hands, lower legs, and on mucocutaneous areas such as the larynx.

c. If untreated, the disease progresses and can involve most organs. Treatment in cases that are chronic and for infection in immunocompromised patients is the administration of amphotericin B, ketoconazole, and itraconazole. If infections of the central nervous system or bone tissue occur, no treatment is effective.

4. Paracoccidioidomycosis

This disease, also called South American blastomycosis, is a chronic, sometimes fatal, disease usually seen in Argentina, Brazil, Columbia, and Venezuela among agricultural workers. It is seldom seen in the United States.

a. Infection occurs via inhalation of airborne mycelial structures of the organism *P. brasiliensis* and produces infection of the respiratory tract that leads to either acute infection, which occurs in children and adolescents; or chronic infection, which occurs in adult men.

b. Lesions appear on the skin, in lymph nodes, and in the lung.

c. Treatment is with itraconazole, sulfadiazine, sulfisoxazole, or amphotericin B.

5. Cryptococcosis

Infection by *Cryptococcus neoformans,* which is found in the soil, particularly soil containing pigeon droppings, causes a subacute chronic infection, involving the lungs, brain, and meninges. Infection results from inhaling aerosolized fungal particles from the environment. The fungus is not dimorphic.

a. The disease, which had been rare, has increased in incidence dramatically. It is the most lethal fungal infection in AIDS patients.

b. AIDS patients, those with Hodgkin's disease, and transplant recipients are at risk for the disease's progressing past the pulmonary phase to disseminated disease. Any organ can be affected. Untreated involvement of the central nervous system is usually fatal.

    c. Treatment for infection-related meningitis is the administration of amphotericin B with flucytosine, but treatment is ineffective in 20% to 30% of these patients.

B. Subcutaneous Mycoses

Most subcutaneous mycoses are the result of puncture wounds with objects contaminated by fungal species found in decaying vegetation and soil.

  1. Sporotrichosis

Infection with *S. schenckii,* which is found in the soil and vegetation, occurs most often among greenhouse workers, farmers, and others who have frequent contact with the soil. Infection is worldwide.

    a. Cutaneous infection produces chronic lesions and infected lymph nodes.

    b. Disseminated disease often involves the skeletal system. Also, inhaled spores can cause pneumonia, especially in immunosuppressed hospitalized patients. Infection mimics tuberculosis.

    c. Treatment of lymphocutaneous infection is with saturated solutions of potassium iodide and itraconazole. Amphotericin B is used in disseminated disease.

  2. Other subcutaneous mycoses are chromoblastomycosis, mycetoma, rhinosporidiosis, lobomycosis, and subcutaneous phycomycosis, all of which produce lesions and are found primarily in tropical and subtropical areas.

C. Cutaneous Mycoses

Fungi that cause diseases of the cutaneous areas of the human body are called dermatophytes. The diseases that they cause are referred to as tineas, or ringworms. These fungi produce enzymes that degrade keratinized tissue, and so can invade epithelial and connective tissues. They do not invade deep tissue. They are found worldwide as saprophytes in the soil, but some of them have evolved to a parasitic existence. Some are strict parasites of human beings. Others are parasitic of animals but can infect human beings also. Some are found free in nature. The cutaneous mycoses are the only contagious fungal diseases in human beings. They can be classified according to the parts of the body in which infection occurs.

  1. Tinea capitis is also referred to as ringworm of the scalp. Infection is caused by species of *Microsporum* and *Tri-*

chophyton. It is transmitted via infected dogs and cats and is usually acquired in childhood.

2. Tinea corporis is an infection of nonhairy areas of the body that is caused by *Trichophyton* and *Microsporum.*

3. Tinea barbae is ringworm of the beard area and can be of two types: superficial infection is caused by *Trichophyticum rubrum;* deeper infections are caused by *Trichophyticum verrucosum,* the result of which is in permanent hair loss.

4. Tinea pedis is ringworm of the feet. Also called athlete's foot, it is caused by many species of the genera *Microsporum, Trichophyton,* and *Epidermophyton.* It is spread primarily through the use of public showers and swimming pools. The infection is aided by failure to completely dry between the toes.

5. Tinea favosa is a second type of ringworm of the scalp that is usually caused by *Trichophyton schoenleinii.* It can cause hair loss.

6. Tinea unguium is a ringworm of the nails. It is of two types: superficial infection that involves only the pits of the nails and significant infection involving the nail surface and invasion beneath the nail plate.

7. Tinea imbricata or ringworm of the torso is caused by *Trichophyticum concentricum* and is restricted to the Pacific Islands, Asia, and Central and South America. It is believed to be transmitted from mother to infant.

8. Tinea cruris is ringworm of the groin, also known as jock itch. It can appear in epidemic form, as the result of exchanging clothing or towels.

9. Treatment of fungal scalp infections is with oral griseofulvin. Body infections are treated with ointments containing 3% salicylic acid, 5% undecylenic acid, 5% benzoic acid, or 5% sodium thiosulfate. Foot infections are treated with ointments containing potassium permanganate, 20% zinc undecylenate, 3% salicylic acid, or 5% benzoic acid. Others drugs include tolnaftate, miconazole nitrate, clotrimazole, and fluconazole.

10. Many dermophytes cause allergic skin reactions that cause vesicular lesions at areas far from the site of infection. These allergic manifestations are referred to as ids.

D. Superficial Mycoses

Infection of the superficial layers of the skin and the hair do not usually require treatment. These infections include tinea versicolor, which causes lesions on the chest, back, and shoulders; tinea nigra palmaris, an asymptomatic infection rarely seen in the United States; piedra black, which affects hair on the scalp, and piedra white, which affects hair of the beard and is seen in immunocompromised patients.

E. Nonpathogenic Organisms

Fungal infections caused by nonpathogenic organisms and that occur in debilitated or traumatized patients or those being treated with broad-spectrum antibiotics or immunosuppressive drugs are referred to as opportunistic fungal infections. Opportunistic fungi are found in the environment as part of normal flora, but any fungus can cause disease in compromised hosts.

1. Candidiasis

Members of the genus *Candida* are found as commensals in animals and human beings in the respiratory tract, intestinal tract, skin, and female genital tract. They are yeasts that under certain circumstances produce pseudohyphae.

a. While most candida infections are endogenous, transmission from mother to fetus and sexual transmission are possible. The species most often involved in infection is *C. albicans*. Others that cause infections are *C. tropicalis, C. parapsilosis, C. glabrata, C. lusitaniae,* and *C. kruesi.*

b. The number of candida infections has increased in recent years as a result of the advent of antibiotics, increased numbers of surgical procedures, and expanded use of immunosuppressive drugs. Infections are either cutaneous or disseminated depending on the condition of the host.

(1) Cutaneous infections occur as the result of conditions such as diabetes, immunological deficiencies, and exposure of the skin to moist environments over a long period. Infections usually produce a superficial epidermatitis.

(2) Disseminated infections are usually iatrogenic (produced by medical care). The administration of some

antibiotics and immunosuppressive drugs discourages the growth of some bacterial species, while the growth of fungal species like *C. albicans* is encouraged. The use of catheters and implantation devices, as well as surgical procedures, provides opportunities for the dissemination of *Candida.*

(3) The virulence of *C. albicans* and related species is the result of several characteristics of the organisms, including the fact that they are dimorphic and convert to the hyphal stage for dissemination in the tissue. They selectively adhere to epithelial and plastic surfaces, can frequently switch among a number of phenotypes, and can release a substance called mannan from their cell walls. Mannan has an immunosuppressive effect.

c. Candida infections are of three clinical types.

(1) Cutaneous infection

(a) One of the most common cutaneous candida infections is oral thrush, in which the tongue is covered by white patches of pseudomembranes composed of fungal cells and epithelium. Thrush is most frequently seen in infants who may acquire the disease from mothers who have vaginal candidiasis. It is also common in AIDS patients. Endogenous thrush is usually the result of taking broad-spectrum antibiotics or immunosuppressive drugs that reduce bacterial flora.

(b) Vaginal candidiasis is associated with diabetes, pregnancy, oral contraceptive use, and antibacterial drugs. Infection causes inflammation of the vagina and produces a thick discharge. Vaginal candidiasis may be the result of deceased numbers of lactobacilli in the vagina resulting from antibiotic therapy. The disease can produce diaper rash in infants. Vaginal candidiasis can be transmitted sexually and in males is called candidal balanitis.

(c) Intertriginous candidiasis affects the feet, hands, groin, axillae, and intergluteal folds, producing lesions of several types. The disease is the result of immersion in water for long periods. Intertriginous candidiasis is also seen in diabetics, obese people, and chronic alcoholics.

(2) Systemic candidiasis is the result of the hematogenous spread of the organism and may affect any organ or tissue including the heart, causing pericarditis, myocarditis, or endocarditis; spinal cord, causing meningitis; and ureters, causing urethritis and cystitis. Infections of the heart can be caused by the use of contaminated needles by heroin addicts, implantation of prosthetic valves, and catheterization with polyethylene catheters. Neonates receiving hyperalimentation therapy or broad-spectrum antibiotics are at risk of candidemia, which can lead to meningitis, arthritis, and osteomyelitis.

(3) Chronic mucocutaneous candidiasis involves the skin, mucous membranes, and any epithelial surface, including the respiratory tract, gastrointestinal tract, and genital epithelium. Infections are associated with immunodeficiency syndromes. Infection usually occurs in infants but may occur in people up to 30 years of age. Fatalities can occur as a result of bacterial sepsis.

(4) Cutaneous infections are treated with creams or powders containing nystatin, gentian violet, or imidazoles. Disseminated candidiasis is treated with amphotericin B, except after kidney transplantation. Flucytosine is used for infections by *C. tropicalis.* Vaginal candidiasis is treated with intravaginal formulations that include butoconazole, clotrimazole, miconazole, tioconazole, and terconazole. Mucocutaneous candidiasis is treated with ketoconazole. Fluconazole is used to treat thrush.

F. Aspergillosis

The genus *Aspergillus,* found in soil, water, decaying vegetation, and any organic debris causes several diseases in human beings. The disease is acquired via inhalation of spores and occurs in both healthy and compromised people. The species *A. fumigatus* most often causes disease, but *A. flavus, A. niger,* and *A. terreus* can also be involved.

1. Allergic aspergillosis

    a. Allergic asthma resulting from exposure to fungal species is a chronic disease, which may become severe. The symptoms include fever, cough, and wheezing induced by the presence of reaginic immunoglobulin E (IgE) antibodies. Spores can germinate within the lungs.

    b. Allergic rhinitis or hay fever can develop as a response to mold spores and mycelia. It may be seasonal or nonseasonal.

    c. Hypersensitivity pneumonitis includes farmers lung, associated with exposure to thermophilic actinomycetes in hay; bagassosis, associated with exposure to bagasse, the residue of sugar cane; and mushroom worker's disease, associated with exposure to mushroom compost. Symptoms last for 12 hours and recovery is spontaneous.

2. Colonizing aspergillosis is a condition that can develop after allergic aspergillosis and is characterized by the formation of a fungus ball, called an aspergilloma, in the lungs. Symptoms are like those of allergic aspergillosis but frequently include hemoptysis.

3. Invasive aspergillosis can develop from either allergic or colonizing disease or can develop independently. The disease is characterized by aspergillus hyphae that penetrate tissue in either a localized or disseminated manner.

    a. Usually, the fungus colonizes the tracheobronchial tree leading to bronchopneumonia and pulmonary hemorrhage, but tissues can also be invaded as the result of hematogenous spread.

    b. At risk for developing invasive disease are renal transplant, leukemia, and lymphoma patients. If untreated, invasive disease is fatal in a matter of weeks.

4. Disseminated aspergillosis can follow invasive disease in patients receiving antimicrobial agents or steroids and occasionally in healthy persons. Many organs are affected, especially the lungs. Death results from bilateral pneumonia or intracerebral hemorrhage.

     5. Invasive disease is treated with amphotericin B, allergic disease is treated with corticosteroids, and lung resection may be necessary for aspergilloma.

  G. Mucormycosis refers to diseases caused by members of the order Mucorales. They are found in the soil, on fruits, and on bread and cause infections in compromised individuals. Infection occurs cutaneously or through inhalation of spores.

     1. When sporangiospores are inhaled and germinate in the nose, severe diseases can result as hyphae spread to the orbit, face, meninges, and frontal lobe of the brain, causing hemorrhage and necrosis. Death can result in a few days after infection, and the overall mortality rate is 50%.

     2. Hyphae that invade the lung cause mass lesions and bronchopneumonia and may spread to the central nervous system. Pulmonary infection occurs most often in patients with uncontrolled leukemia.

     3. Cutaneous mucormycosis occurs in patients who have experienced trauma or who have had contaminated bandages applied to wounds.

  H. Pneumocystis pneumonia is an infection caused by *P. carinii,* which is widely found in nature as a saprophyte in the lungs of human beings and animals.

     1. It causes pneumonia in premature, malnourished infants, patients receiving corticosteroids, and in over 80% of AIDS patients. Symptoms include fever, nonproductive cough, and shortness of breath.

     2. Bronchoalveolar lavage and transtracheal lung biopsy are frequently necessary for diagnosis. Treatment is with trimethoprim-sulfamethoxazole or dapsone and aerosolized and intravenous pentamidine.

  I. Mycotoxins

    Mushroom poisoning, referred to as mycetismus, results from the ingestion of various poisonous, fleshy, field fungi, especially those of the genus *Amanita.* One or two hours after ingestion, symptoms including profuse sweating, severe gastritis, diarrhea, and convulsions appear. Death may occur within 12 hours.

  J. Mycotoxicosis is the result of metabolites produced by fungi when they grow on foods or grains. Aflatoxin B_1 is believed to cause liver cancer when contaminated grains are stored for long periods before ingestion, especially in the Far East and India, but mycotoxins have also been found in peanut butter in the United States.

XVI. Parasites

In this section, the term parasite refers to animal (extracellular) parasites (see I, B, 1). Animal parasites spend at least part of their lives in the human body.

A. Animal parasites include the Protozoa, or single-cell animal parasites; the Nemathelminthes, or roundworms; the Platyhelminthes, or flatworms; and the Arthropoda, or invertebrate animals with jointed appendages.

B. Worldwide, the cost of parasitic infection in human terms is enormous. In 1990, malaria caused between one and two million deaths, schistosomiasis caused 200 000 deaths, and amebiasis caused up to 110 000 deaths. In the United States, epidemics of parasitic infections are caused by protozoa when sanitation procedures fail. Some parasites enter the country via immigrants. Parasitic infections are often seen in compromised hosts, e.g., AIDS patients.

C. The incidence of parasitic infections is associated with the climate, the availability of hosts and vector, the dietary and sanitary habits of populations, the mode of dress, and the nutritional status of hosts.

D. The stages in parasitic development are called its life cycles, during which parasites often exist in different forms such as sporozoites or cysts, eggs, and larval forms. They usually cause disease in their adult forms.

E. Parasites may live in several hosts during their life cycles. Intermediate hosts are those in which parasites develop but do not reach maturity. Definitive hosts are those in which parasites reach maturity. Many intermediate hosts may be involved in a life cycle before a parasite reaches its definitive host.

F. Parasites harm human beings in many different ways. They cause cell destruction, either physically or chemically; they may rob hosts of nutrition; or they cause physical trauma. Many parasites, however, exist in hosts without causing symptoms or overt disease.

XVII. The Protozoa

The groups of parasitic protozoa are Sarcodina, Mastigophora, Ciliata, and Sporozoa.

A. Sarcodina (*Amoeba*)

Several groups of the *Amoeba* exist in the human intestinal tract as commensals (see I. A), but *Entamoeba histolytica* causes amebiasis and amebic dysentery by invading the tissue of the intestinal tract. It is believed that there are two forms of *E. histolytica,* one that is pathogenic, and one that is not.

1. Although most infections with *E. histolytica* are asymptomatic, patients who are symptomatic develop either intestinal or extraintestinal pathology.

   a. Intestinal disease produces abdominal pain and frequent bowel movements. Invasive intestinal disease (of the colon) produces gradual development of abdominal pain, diarrhea, dysentery, and weight loss. If the colon is invaded, ulcers develop. The result is necrosis and violent dysentery with bloody mucus and, often, secondary bacterial infections that have a high mortality rate.

   b. Extraintestinal disease is the result of intestinal invasion by trophozoites (the active, vegetative stage of protozoons), which are carried to the liver via circulating blood. Other organs that can become involved are the lungs, pericardium, brain, and skin.

2. Human beings are the major reservoir for *E. histolytica,* with 480 million people currently infected and carrying the organism, though only 10% develop symptoms. Infection occurs via ingestion of food or liquids that are contaminated with *E. histolytica* cysts from human feces or from direct fecal-oral contact. The use of untreated water and the use of human feces as fertilizer are the major causes of dissemination of the organism. Groups at risk are travelers, immigrants, migrant workers, and active male homosexuals.

3. Symptomatic intestinal disease is treated with metronidazole and iodoquinol. Extraintestinal disease is treated with metronidazole, dehydroemetine, and chloroquine. Asymptomatic cyst passers are treated with diloxanide furoate. However, control of infection is dependent on proper hygiene, sanitation, and education.

4. Primary amebic meningoencephalitis is caused by *Naegleria fowleri,* an organism that can transform into a flagellate and has been found in soil, water, cooling towers, sewage sludge, hospital hydrothermal pools, and swimming pools. Most infections have been associated with the practice of swimming in warm fresh water. Infection occurs when trophozoites enter the nasal cavity via inhalation of contaminated dust or aspiration of water. Following an incubation period of 3 to 15 days, the organism travels from the olfactory bulbs to the central nervous system, causing hemorrhages in the cerebral tissue. Symptoms include severe headache, fever, nausea and vomiting, encephalitis, seizures, and coma. Infection usually causes death in 7 to 10 days. No effective treatment for the disease exists.

5. *Acanthamoeba,* found in well water, dust, and soil, have caused infections of the skin, respiratory tract, and corneas via contaminated air, water, and contact lenses. In debilitated patients, infection can spread to the central nervous system resulting in chronic amoebic encephalitis. Effects of the disease include skin ulcers, liver disease, pneumonitis, pharyngitis, and renal failure. Symptoms include fever, headache, stiff neck, altered mental status, paresis, lethargy, and coma. Fatalities are usually the result of eventual bronchopneumonia.

B. Mastigophora

Members of the class Mastigophora develop flagella and/or undulating membranes that enable them to propel themselves.

1. *Giardia lamblia* is a flagellated protozoan that causes giardiasis, an intestinal disease suffered by travelers worldwide. In the United States it is seen in people who drink contaminated water, in children in day-care centers, and in homosexual males.

a. Infection is the result of the ingestion of cysts that pass unharmed to the duodenum where trophozoites are produced. After 2 weeks, the symptoms of low-grade fever, nausea, and severe watery diarrhea develop and last 3 to 4 days.

b. Chronic infection may develop causing intermittent diarrhea for more than 2 years. Other symptoms of chronic infection are headache, myalgia, weight loss, anorexia, and malabsorption syndrome, which is an interference with absorption of fats and carbohydrates.

c. Although human beings are the main reservoir for the parasite, it has been found in beavers, muskrats, and water moles. Campers and backpackers who drink untreated stream water are also at risk for the disease.

d. Treatment of the disease is the administration of metronidazole, quinacrine, and furazolidone. Ingestion of potentially contaminated water should be preceded by boiling the water for one minute or mixing 2 to 4 drops of household bleach or 0.5 ml of 2% tincture of iodine to each liter of water, and putting it aside for one hour before drinking.

2. *Trichomonas* species or *T. vaginalis* causes vaginitis in women and urethritis or prostatitis in men as well as asymptomatic infection in both sexes. The symptoms of infection in women are a thick yellow, blood-tinged discharge, with burning or itching sensations. In men, the symptoms are painful urination or no symptoms. Treatment is with metronidazole orally and/or by vaginal suppositories.

3. African trypanosomiasis, or sleeping sickness, is caused by *Trypanosoma* species, *T. brucei gambiense,* and *T. brucei rhodesiense* via the bite of the tsetse fly.

    a. Several days after the infection, episodes of parasitemia occur, causing headaches, joint pain, malaise, and enlarged lymph nodes and spleen.

    b. The sleeping sickness stage of the disease involves the central nervous system. It causes insomnia, irritability, personality changes, and loss of central nervous system function.

    c. Advanced disease produces convulsion, coma, and death from malnutrition and secondary infection. *T. brucei rhodesiense* infections last weeks to months, *T. brucei gambiense* infections last months to years.

    d. *T. brucei rhodesiense* and *gambiense* are transmitted to human beings via tsetse flies. *T. brucei rhodesiense* is harbored in wild game and domestic animals, but *T. brucei gambiense* is thought to exist only in human beings and tsetse flies.

    e. Treatment of Gambian sleeping sickness is with the administration of eflornithine. Rhodesian disease is treated with suramin and pentamidine.

4. *T. cruzi,* the cause of American trypanosomiasis, or Chagas' disease, is harbored in human beings; domesticated animals, including cats and dogs; and in wild animals. The disease is transmitted via the bite of the reduviid bug, called the assassin bug or kissing bug in the United States. Transmission can also be via blood transfusions. The disease causes 50 000 deaths per year in Latin America. Two forms of the disease occur.

   a. Acute disease produces lymphadenopathy near the site of the insect bite, and symptoms are mild and self-limiting, but in some cases infection can result in acute meningoencephalitis or myocarditis.

   b. Chronic disease causes heart enlargement and congestive heart failure.

   c. Treatment is administration of nifurtimox and benznidazole.

5. Sandflies are the vectors that disseminate the species of *Leishmania* that cause leishmaniasis worldwide in warm climates.

   a. In cutaneous leishmaniasis, sores develop at each area of insect bite and may become secondarily infected.

   b. In mucocutaneous disease, infection at the original site of infection spreads to the nasal and oral mucosa, causing extensive erosive lesions.

   c. In visceral disease, also known as kalaazar, infection results in the enlargement of the spleen, lymph nodes, lungs, and digestive tract.

   d. Treatment is with antimony sodium gluconate or N-methylglucamine.

C. Ciliata

   Balantidium coli is the largest and only ciliated protozoan that is pathogenic to human beings. Human infection is rare even though the organism is harbored in 60% to 90% of hogs. The chief symptom of infection is diarrhea, and treatment is with iodoquinol and oxytetracycline.

D. Sporozoa

   The sporozoa have complex life cycles that include both sexual and asexual generations. The most important genera to man are *Plasmodium.*

   1. Malaria, also called plasmodiasis, malaria is caused by four species of *Plasmodium: P. falciparum* (malignant ter-

tian malaria), *P. vivax* (benign tertian malaria), *P. malariae* (quartan malaria), and *P. ovale* (ovale malaria). Acute malaria develops in 3 million people each year, and 1 million African children die from the disease annually.

  a. The two important phases of the life cycle of the malarial parasite are

- Sporogony, or the sexual phase, which occurs in the female *Anopheles* mosquito
- Schizogony, or the nuclear division of the organism, which takes place in the primate or human host

  b. Within an infected individual, malarial attacks occur in cycles in conjunction with the release of merozoites (a form of the organism) in the bloodstream, e.g., in tertian malaria, the attacks occur every 48 hours.

  c. Symptoms during attacks are chills lasting 15 to 60 minutes, headache, nausea, vomiting, temperatures of 105°F or higher, and profuse sweating. Infection may be asymptomatic, severe, or fatal.

  d. Treatment for prophylaxis, suppression of an attack, or prevention of attack in an infected person is through the administration of chloroquine, and primaquine phosphate, mefloquine, and quinine for *P. falciparum* infections.

2. Toxoplasmosis is a disease that can be acquired by both healthy and immunocompromised people and is caused by *Toxoplasma gondii* for which members of the cat family are hosts. The organisms are shed into the environment through the feces of the animal where they cause the infection of other warm-blooded animals, such as cattle. Plants can also be contaminated.

  a. Human infection occurs through handling of contaminated raw meat, ingestion of incompletely cooked meat, handling of litter boxes, gardening without gloves, and inadequate washing of home-grown vegetables.

  b. Human infections are usually asymptomatic but lymphadenopathy and hepatosplenomegaly can develop, as well as reactivation disease in immunosuppressed individuals, AIDS patients, or those with cancer of the lymphatic system.

c. Reactivation of infection often leads to disseminated disease. In AIDS patients, the sites affected are the central nervous system and the lungs, which often produce fatalities.

d. The disease can be acquired transplacentally if a mother has a primary infection during pregnancy. Less than 1% of infants develop pathology, but infection can cause severe mental retardation and visual handicaps.

e. Treatment of infection is with pyrimethamine and sulfadiazine.

3. Babesiosis, also referred to as Nantucket fever, is a malaria-like illness caused by *Babesia microti,* which is transmitted to human beings via the same tick that is the primary vector in Lyme disease. It can also be acquired via blood transfusions. Hosts involved in the life cycle of the organism are the white-footed mouse and the white-tailed deer. The disease produces prolonged fever and anemia, and varies in severity from inapparent, subclinical infection to fatal disease. Treatment is the administration of clindamycin and quinine.

4. Several cryptosporidium organisms cause gastrointestinal disease that include waterborne epidemics, traveler's diarrhea, day-care center outbreaks, disease in immunocompromised individuals, and disease in animals. The disease is transmitted to human beings via ingestion of water that is contaminated by the feces of farm animals, mice, birds, and other animals. In day-care center disease, children younger than 3, who are in diapers and who are not toilet trained, are usually involved. Treatment is nonspecific, but included are the use of antidiarrheal agents, nutritional management, and the administration of fluids.

XVIII. The Nemathelminthes

Members of the phylum Nemathelminthes are nonsegmented oval worms with well-developed digestive tracts. Separate individual organisms are male or female.

A. Ascariasis, or roundworm infection, is caused by *Ascaris lumbricoides.* These organisms resemble earthworms and invade the intestinal tracts of human beings. Adult worms are 8 to 12 inches long.

1. *A. lumbricoides* is found throughout the world, and it infects approximately one billion people.

2. Fecal contamination and use of human feces as fertilizer creates areas of endemic infection where virtually everyone harbors the worm. Each female worm produces 200 000 eggs per day, and eggs remain viable in the soil for as long as 10 years.

3. Infection is the result of contact with contaminated soil or the ingestion of contaminated food. Ingested eggs hatch in the duodenum and are transported via the blood to the lungs where they cause hemorrhage and infection. This can result in a pneumonitis or asthma-like response. The larvae then move up the respiratory tree and are swallowed. The adult worms develop in the intestine where they cause minor symptoms in adults but toxic symptoms or intestinal obstruction in children.

4. Treatment is with mebendazole or pyrantel pamoate. Intestinal obstruction requires surgery.

5. Visceral larva migrans involves nematodes that migrate through the human body, usually in children between the ages of 1 and 5 who have contact with pets or who have pica. Infection can involve the lungs, eyes, or other organs.

B. Hookworm infection is caused by *Necator americanus* (New World hookworm) or *Ancylostoma duodenale* (Old World hookworm), and infection is via contact with contaminated soil, rocks, or grass.

1. Infection causes anemia and loss of proteins. Severe or repetitive infections, especially in children, can cause both physical retardation and mental retardation.

2. In the United States hookworm infection occurs primarily on the Atlantic coast, though infection is now unusual. Treatment is with mebendazole and the correction of malnutrition, including iron loss. The wearing of footwear decreases the incidence of disease.

C. Cutaneous larva migrans is caused by dog and cat hookworm species that penetrate the human skin, most often the skin of children, farmers, and others who have contact with the soil, particularly where dogs and cats have defecated. The larvae burrow into subcutaneous tissue causing conditions referred to as serpiginous dermatitis, creeping eruption, or ground itch, which can lead to secondary bacterial infections. Treatment is with topical applications of thiabendazole.

D. Strongyloidiasis is caused by *Strongyloides stercoralis,* which penetrates intact human skin while in its larval form. Infection involves the liver, kidneys, brain, lymph nodes, cutaneous and subcutaneous tissues, and may be fatal. The disease is found primarily in warm, moist, tropical climates worldwide and in the rural southern United States. Treatment is the administration of thiabendazole, antibiotics, and intravenous fluids.

E. Enterobiasis, called pinworm or seatworm infection, is caused by *Enterobiasis vermicularis,* which are yellowish-white worms 2 to 13 mm long. Adult worms inhabit the cecum, ileum, and appendix, causing mild inflammation. Perianal itching results, usually during the night as the female worms leave the anus to deposit eggs in the perianal area. This can cause a person to scratch the area, leading to secondary bacterial infections as well as the spread of worm infection to other people via hands and articles such as bedding and clothing. Infection is found worldwide, primarily in children 5 to 9 years of age. Treatment through the administration of mebendazole and pyrantel pamoate is effective, but reinfections are common.

F. Trichinosis, or muscle-worm infection, is caused by *Trichinella spiralis* and is the result of ingesting live, encysted larvae in meat. There are three phases of the disease.

1. As the larvae mature into adults in the duodenum and produce more larvae in the intestinal wall, the symptoms of diarrhea, abdominal discomfort, and vomiting occur.

2. As the larvae enter the capillaries and lymphatics from the intestine and migrate through the lungs, heart, and systemic circulation, infection, particularly striated muscle tissue as well as symptoms of periorbital swelling, fever, myalgia, and rash occur.

3. As the larvae become encysted in striated muscle, sometimes the heart and central nervous system, the symptoms of muscle pain, weakness, and cachexia (wasting) develop.

4. Although trichinosis was once a common worm infection in the United States caused by ingestion of contaminated

pork, beef, and wild game, the incidence has decreased greatly as a result of public education, the use of deep freezers, and the decrease of infection in swine.

5. Since there is no satisfactory treatment for trichinosis, care in cooking pork is still essential, since only 70% of pork products are processed through federally inspected firms and even that is inspected only for contamination visible to the naked eye. Infections have been traced to small meat-packing firms and homemade sausage. Smoking, spicing, salting, pickling, and drying of meats (pork or pork mixtures) cannot be relied upon to destroy trichinae. Pork must be cooked until no pinkness remains and it reaches an internal temperature of 137°F.

6. Filariasis is a group of infectious diseases caused by arthropod-borne nematodes, usually in India and the South Pacific. Infection occurs as the result of the bite of infected arthropods, such as mosquitoes and flies. Infection of lymphatics and subcutaneous tissue occurs and usually results in symptomatic disease after repeated or heavy infection. This is referred to as lymphatic filariasis, which can lead to elephantiasis or tropical pulmonary eosinophilia. Ocular disease resulting from *Onchocerca volvulus*, referred to as river blindness, is one of the leading preventable causes of blindness worldwide. Treatment of all types of filariasis is with diethylcarbamazine citrate.

XIX. The Platyhelminthes

Flatworms are bilaterally symmetrical and appear flat. Most are hermaphroditic. Two classes cause infection in human beings.

A. Trematoda are classified according to the organ in which the adult form is found.

1. Liver, intestinal, and lung flukes are leaf shaped and attach to organs by means of ventral suckers. They have complex life cycles and use snails and crustacea as intermediate hosts.

2. Infection is usually via ingestion of raw or poorly cooked fish, crabs, crayfish, and aquatic plants.

3. Blood flukes cause schistosomiasis, a disease in which *Schistosoma mansoni* infect human beings as the result of contact with contaminated fresh water. This is known as dermatitis and swimmer's itch. Chronic schistosomiasis

causes granulomatous disease involving primarily the liver and spleen. A disease that occurs worldwide, schistosomiasis infects about 400 000 people in the United States, many of whom are Puerto Ricans. Transmission is not believed to be a problem in the United States because sanitation conditions are good and the appropriate snail hosts are unavailable. Treatment is with praziquantel.

B. Cestoidea are ribbonlike worms known as tapeworms that invade the intestines but occasionally other organs as well. They are actually chains of organisms with a head that anchors to the intestinal mucosa. The number of segments varies from a few to thousands. Tapeworms have no digestive systems and so rely on absorption to gain nutrients from their hosts.

1. Taeniasis is an infection caused by the genus *Taenia*. *Taenia solium* is the pork tapeworm and *Taenia saginata* is the beef tapeworm. Infections with adult tapeworms are not usually serious, but infection with tapeworm larvae can be serious.

a. *T. solium* infects human beings as its definitive hosts, and pigs are infected as a result of eating material contaminated by human feces. Human beings are then infected by eating cyst-bearing pork.

b. If, however, human beings ingest *T. solium* ova via food, drink, or fingers contaminated with human feces, human cysticercosis can occur in which larval cysts appear in any organ but usually in the central nervous system, eye, and skeletal muscle. Symptoms include epilepsy, mental disturbances, and reduction in visual acuity.

c. Treatment is with praziquantel but surgery may be necessary.

2. Echinococcosis genera are the smallest of the tapeworms that infect human beings. Most infections are caused by *Echinococcus granulosus,* which is parasitic in dogs, sheep, and cattle. Human beings are usually only accidental hosts as the result of exposure to contaminated feces. Cysts can form in any organ but usually the liver and lungs are involved. If cysts leak and the organism enters the bloodstream, allergic symptoms, edema, asthma, and anaphylactic shock can result. Fatalities are not unusual. Treatment is the surgical removal of a single cyst; multiple cysts are treated with mebendazole.

XX. The Arthropoda

Most arthropods that are important to human disease are in the classes Insecta and Arachnia.

A. Arthropods have at some stage in their life cycles, paired, jointed appendages, a chitinized exoskeleton, and a body cavity through which bloodlike fluid circulates.

B. Included in Insecta (having three pairs of walking legs) are flies, fleas, lice, bees, and wasps.

C. Arthropods' life cycles include stages referred to as instars (between moltings), nymphs, larvae, pupa, and adults.

D. Arthropods affect human beings as ectoparasites, as intermediate or definitive hosts of other animal parasites, as venom-producing agents, and as vectors of infectious disease.

E. Arthropods that cause the spread of disease while feeding or living on the human skin include the itch mite, fleas, ticks, bedbugs, kissing bugs, body lice, and maggots.

F. As vectors, arthropods spread bacterial, viral, rickettsial, and mycotic disease in human beings.

SUGGESTED READING

Baron, S., ed. *Medical Microbiology,* 3d ed. New York: Churchill Livingstone, 1991.

Belows, A., ed. *Manual of Clinical Microbiology.* Washington, D.C.: American Society for Microbiology, 1991.

Boyd, R. F. *Basic Medical Microbiology,* 5th ed. Boston: Little, Brown, 1995.

Centers for Disease Control. "Case-Control Study of HIV Seroconversion in Health-Care Workers after Percutaneous Exposure to HIV-Infected Blood—France, United Kingdom, and United States." *Morbidity and Mortality Weekly Report* 44 (1995): 929–933.

Hoeprich, P. D., M. C. Jordan, and A. R. Ronald. *Infectious Diseases,* 5th ed. Philadelphia: J.B. Lippincott, 1994.

Howard, B. J. *Clinical and Pathogenic Microbiology,* 2d ed. St. Louis: Mosby-Yearbook, 1994.

Chapter 4

Scientific Bases of Sterilization and Disinfection

CHAPTER OBJECTIVES

Upon completion of this chapter, the reader will be able to

1. compare and contrast the concepts of sterilization and disinfection
2. compare and contrast steam autoclaving and pasteurization
3. discuss the disadvantage of using ethyl and isopropyl alcohol for disinfection
4. describe the importance of surfactants in the control of microorganisms
5. discuss the advantages and disadvantages of using glutaraldehyde as a sterilizing-disinfecting agent
6. list the precautions necessary for the safe use of ethylene oxide gas from both the patient's and practitioner's points of view

Knowledge of proper sterilization and disinfection procedures is essential for respiratory therapists to perform their jobs safely and effectively. The nature of the procedures we perform is such that a therapist who is not knowledgeable in this area can expose patients to a myriad of potentially lethal diseases. A proper understanding of these procedures and the necessary equipment and chemicals used includes knowledge of the scientific principles on which they are based.

I. Definitions

A. *Sterile* means "absence of viable forms of microorganisms." Sterilization destroys or removes all microorganisms, both vegetative and spore forms. There are no degrees of sterility. An object cannot be "almost sterile." If any viable (alive) microorganisms are present, the object may be clean, but it is not sterile.

B. *Disinfection* refers to the process of destroying by the use of either chemical agents or physical means at least the pathogenic organisms that are in the vegetative state. A disinfected object is not sterile and is not expected to be sterile. Disinfection is carried out on inanimate objects.

C. *Antisepsis* is the process in which the destruction of pathogenic organisms in the vegetative state is accomplished on living tissue, e.g., the skin. Because tissue is sensitive to chemical and physical disinfecting procedures, such as boiling and other techniques, disinfecting techniques cannot be used for the purpose of antisepsis.

D. *Degermation* is the process of removing microorganisms, especially transients, from the skin by the use of chemicals (soaps, antiseptics) and mechanical action (scrubbing).

E. *Sanitation* is the process of reducing the number of microorganisms on inanimate objects to the level of public health standards, e.g., food service items.

F. Agents with the suffix "-static" prevent the multiplication of the organism named in the prefix, e.g., a bacteriostat prevents the multiplication of bacteria.

G. Agents with the suffix "-cidal" kill the form of microorganism named in the prefix, e.g., sporicidal agents kill spores.

II. Environmental Factors in Sterilization and Disinfection

A. Improper Handling

Regardless of the efforts made to destroy pathogenic microorganisms, if the objects or areas that have been treated are then improperly handled, the efforts are void.

B. Heat Sensitivity

There is no one sterilization or disinfection method that is universally applicable. Of all the methods for destroying pathogenic microbes, heat is the most effective. But many things that must be treated cannot be exposed to extreme heat, e.g., delicate instruments, gauges.

C. Interfering Matter

Before any attempt to sterilize or disinfect an item is made, all soil must be removed because it interferes with the sterilization-disinfection process. In the health care field, soil is usually organic matter such as mucus, blood, saliva, or feces. Lubricants often present on medical instruments also are a form of soil and must be removed.

III. Physical Methods of Sterilization and Disinfection

A. Moist Heat

Moist heat is an effective method of killing microorganisms. Vegetative forms of bacteria, yeasts, molds, and most viruses are killed in 5 to 10 minutes at 80°C. Mold spores are killed in 30 minutes at 80°C. Bacterial spores require moist heat for at least 15 minutes at 121°C for destruction. Moist heat kills microorganisms through the coagulation of their proteins, but other changes caused by moist heat, such as inactivation of enzymes, changes in nucleic acids, and cytoplasmic membrane aberrations, also contribute to the organism's death.

B. Boiling

Boiling is not reliably sporicidal but can be used for disinfection as vegetative forms of infectious agents are killed in 30 minutes at sea level.

C. Steam

Steam at atmospheric pressure is much hotter than boiling water. At 100°C it has 540 calories of heat versus 180 calories of boiling water at 100°C. This heat is released when the steam condenses on a cooler surface.

D. Steam Autoclaving

Steam autoclaving is done under pressure (Figure 4–1). Although steam is much hotter than boiling water, the amount of time necessary to kill spores with steam at 100°C is impractical. In order to raise the temperature of steam, it is placed under a pressure of 15 pounds per square inch (psi), which raises the temperature to 121°C. Virtually all spores are killed when steam at 121°C is applied for 15 minutes. If the pressure is increased to 20 psi, the temperature rises to 126°C, and virtually all spores are killed in 10 minutes. Moist heat sterilization is performed in a sealed chamber called an autoclave and is the preferred method of sterilization when possible. A request that an item be autoclaved is the equivalent to a request that it be sterilized (Figure 4–1).

1. The purpose of autoclaving items is, for all practical purposes, to sterilize them. But the fact that something has

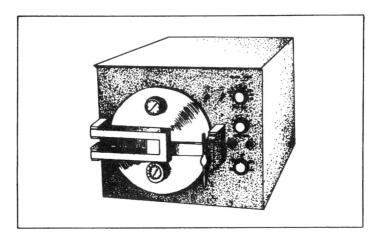

Figure 4–1 Tabletop Autoclave for Small Loads.

been autoclaved does not mean that it is sterile. Several things are necessary for sterility to be achieved.

a. The items must be properly wrapped and placed within the autoclave so that the steam can reach all surfaces of the item. Wrapping materials include muslin, linen cloth, craft paper, brown paper, crêpe paper, Mylar, and vegetable parchment.

b. The proper temperature must be achieved for the proper length of time.

c. All air in the autoclave must be replaced by steam.

d. At the end of the cycle, the autoclave must be properly vented. Loads that contain liquids must be vented slowly or the liquids will boil and burst their containers.

2. The proof of successful autoclaving involves the placement of indicators in the autoclave load so that the sterility of the load can be checked.

a. Chemical indicators are specially treated tape or bags that change color at 121°C (Figure 4–2).

b. Biological sterilization indicators (Figure 4–3) are capsules containing a strip impregnated with bacterial spores, pH indicators, and a culture medium in a crushable am-

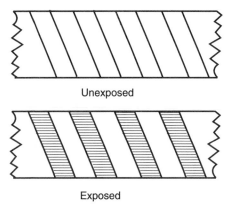

Unexposed

Exposed

Figure 4–2 Chemical Indicator Tape, before and after Exposure.

pule. After autoclaving, the ampule is crushed, and the color of the strip is checked. Spores of *B. stearothermophilus* are most often used in biological indicators. Spores of other species are used for different sterilization processes such as dry heat or ethylene oxide. They are chosen for their susceptibility to each procedure.

c. Culture tests or biological monitors are the most reliable indicators of sterilization; however, they require an incubation period before they can be assessed.

d. The Joint Commission and Communicable Disease Center recommend that steam autoclaves be tested once a week with spore indicators.

e. Thermocouples are inserted into the autoclave load to monitor temperature during sterilization. The temperature throughout the process is recorded.

E. Pasteurization

Pasteurization is a physical method of disinfection, not sterilization, and is most widely used in the processing of food. Beer, wine, and milk are examples of liquids that are pasteurized during their preparation. Pasteurization employs the application of mild heat to destroy vegetative pathogenic organisms. Two techniques may be used in this process.

1. The batch method, or holding method, is the process in which heat is applied at 62.0°C for 30 minutes. Medical

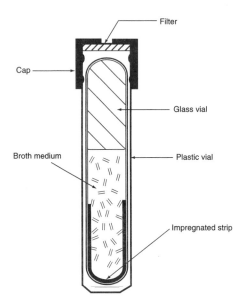

Figure 4–3 Biological Sterilization Indicator.

---

equipment pasteurizers such as those used to disinfect respiratory therapy equipment operate at this temperature.
2. The flash method is used to pasteurize milk. Milk is run as a thin film over pipes held at 71.7°C for a period of 15 seconds.
F. Dry Heat
Some materials cannot be sterilized or disinfected by any wet-heat method because they would be adversely affected by the water. Powders and oils are such products. Dry heat is the method used to eliminate pathogenic microorganisms from these materials. Since microorganisms, especially spores, are much less susceptible to dry heat than they are to wet heat, higher temperatures, in the range of 160°C to 180°C, must be applied for a period of 1 to 2 hours. The air in the ovens must be mechanically circulated in order to ensure even distribution of the heat. The microorganisms are destroyed as a result of oxidation, desiccation, and changes in osmotic pressures.
G. Incineration
Disposable, combustible equipment and supplies that have been contaminated are best treated by the method of incineration. Most disposable equipment and needles are not designed

to be effectively sterilized for reuse. Often the material of which they are made will not tolerate conventional hospital sterilizing methods and so should be disposed of by burning after a single use. Flaming is a process used to kill microorganisms by exposing heat-tolerant items to a direct flame. Flaming has no application for respiratory therapy equipment.

H. Filtration

Two substances that are particularly difficult to sterilize or disinfect are liquids and gases. Sterilization and/or disinfection of liquids and gases is accomplished through the process of filtration. The sterilization and/or disinfection of medical gases in the hospital is primarily the responsibility of respiratory care practitioners who are responsible for providing uncontaminated gases to patients through therapeutic devices. There are three types of filters used for this purpose.

1. Copper bead filters are placed in ventilators and other equipment by the manufacturers to prevent physical debris from entering the equipment through compressed gas sources. They are usually located at the point where compressed gas enters the device.

2. Membrane filters are very thin sheets of sievelike, inert cellulose esters and other polymeric materials. Those used in respiratory care are usually folded over many times to provide a large surface area of filter material within a small canister. The filters are constructed so that they are most effective when the gas is passed through them in one particular direction. The proper direction is indicated on the filter canister. Filters may be autoclavable or disposable. Manufacturers' instructions must be followed regarding their testing and reuse. Some of these filters are effective against viruses.

3. High-efficiency particulate air (HEPA) filters remove particles as small as 0.3 μm from the air with 99.97% efficiency. They are used in high-flow air control systems to remove physical particles including microorganisms. They are also used in burn rooms and in biohazard hoods.

I. Ultrasonic Cleaners

High-frequency sound waves sent through a solution are very efficient in removing soil from immersed equipment. Electric energy is converted to physical energy by piezoelectric transducers that produce a phenomenon called cavitation within the solution. The physical energy causes tiny bubbles to form in the solution, and the collapse of the bubbles produces a suction effect that removes soil. Ultrasonic cleaners are used primarily as pasteurizers that remove interfering organic matter prior to sterilization.

J. Radiation Disinfection
    There are two types of electromagnetic radiation that affect microorganisms, and they have different applications.
    1. Ultraviolet Radiation
        Ultraviolet (UV) rays are effective in sterilizing and disinfecting because they produce photochemical reactions in microbial DNA. The use of UV lamps, referred to as germicidal lamps, aids in reducing the number of microorganisms in the air, i.e., in nurseries. The wavelength most commonly used is 2537 A. Since warm air normally rises, carrying microorganisms with it, the lamps are usually positioned to reflect upwardly. Ultraviolet rays are also used in the sterilization of vaccines and toxins, as well as in the food-packaging industry. The disadvantages of UV radiation are that it has little penetrating power, and overexposure to UV radiation causes skin erythema and conjunctivitis.

K. Ionizing Radiation
    Shorter wavelength electromagnetic rays are extremely effective in sterilizing and are used extensively by the manufacturers of medical supplies. The two types of short-wavelength electromagnetic rays include X-rays, which are produced by electron generators, and gamma rays, which are produced by the decay of radioactive substances. There are two theories about the method in which this radiation affects microorganisms. The first is that the atoms of DNA are damaged, and the other is that the destruction is accomplished through ionization of the cells' water, which in turn produces powerful oxidizing and reducing agents within the cell. Many products used by respiratory therapists are prepackaged and have been sterilized by this method. Such packages must be thoroughly checked for damage before use.

IV. **Chemical Methods of Sterilization and Disinfection**

Certain chemicals called chemosterilizers or sterilants can be used to achieve sterility under certain conditions. They destroy pathogenic microorganisms through cell membrane injury, coagulation, denaturation, interaction with groups of proteins, and/or oxidation. There are several groups of chemicals used for sterilization and disinfection.

A. Phenol and Phenolics

Phenol was the disinfectant used by Joseph Lister to show the beneficial effects of killing pathogenic microorganisms in the operating room. At that time, it was called carbolic acid. Phenolics, phenol derivatives, phenol-related compounds, and phenol homologues are all derived from phenol. They are unusually active in the presence of organic matter, stay active on surfaces long after application, become reactivated when rehydrated, and are tuberculocidal.

1. Hexachlorophene

Hexachlorophene was a very popular disinfectant in hospitals for a number of years, especially for hand washing, because it provided a long, low level of antimicrobial activity. Since 1972 the use of this chemical has been severely restricted, and it is now a prescription item. It was shown to be absorbed by the skin and caused brain damage in premature infants washed with hexachlorophene soap.

2. Other phenolics

The principal remaining phenolic is chloroprene, but several others are important in general sanitation.

B. Alcohols

Ethyl and isopropyl alcohol are the only alcohols that are extensively used. Others are more effective but are not used because of their unpleasant odors. Ethyl and isopropyl alcohols are equally effective and are best used in a 70% concentration. Aqueous alcohol is more effective than absolute alcohol. Both ethyl and isopropyl alcohols are bactericidal, tuberculocidal, and fungicidal but not sporicidal. Enveloped viruses are also susceptible to alcohols. They have high antimicrobial activity levels on environmental surfaces.

C. Halogens (Inorganic Halogen Compounds)

Chlorine and iodine are the halogens in common use, although others are utilized as antimicrobial agents in other disinfectants.

1. Chlorine

Elemental and inorganic chlorine are used for sanitation, water purification, and disinfection. Organic matter severely interferes with chlorine's antimicrobial activity.

Hypochlorites are used as bleaching agents and sanitizing agents in dairies, meat processing facilities, and swimming pools. Sodium hypochlorite (household bleach) is an effective germicide diluted 1:10 to 1:100 depending on the amount of interfering matter that is present. It should be prepared daily for use as a germicide. It is corrosive to some metals, especially aluminum.

2. Iodine

Tinctures of iodine, which are simply iodine dissolved in alcohol, are the most popular agents for wound and skin antisepsis and are also used as general disinfectants and in water purification. Tinctures of 1%, 5%, and 7% destroy skin bacteria in 90, 60, and 15 seconds respectively. Their disadvantages are that in strong concentrations they cause tissue necrosis, they leave stains, and some people are allergic to them.

3. Iodophors

Iodophors are composed of iodine and surface-active organic carrier molecules. Although their antimicrobial activity is not as great as that of the tinctures, they are nonstaining, nonallergenic, water soluble, and relatively nonirritating.

D. Surfactants

Surfactants are used principally for the reduction of surface tension. Even though they are not antimicrobial, they are invaluable in the control of microorganisms.

1. Soaps

Most soaps are sodium and potassium salts of higher fatty acids. When used on the skin, they emulsify the oily layer where most transient microorganisms are present. Washing with a soap mechanically removes microorganisms. Many cosmetic soaps contain bacteriostatic or bactericidal compounds.

2. Detergents

Detergents are synthetic cleaning agents that have a surfactant effect. They do not form precipitates with water minerals as soaps do.

a. Anionic detergents are utilized in laundry powders and liquids. They mechanically remove soil from articles, but they are not disinfectants.

b. Cationic detergents contain ions of ammonium, phosphonium, sulfonium, and other "onium" ions, including the quaternary ammonium ion compounds called the "quats." They are effective agents against a broad spectrum of vegetative cells and enveloped viruses but have limited sporicidal or virucidal effectiveness. They are bland, nontoxic, and inexpensive, but they have many serious disadvantages. They are not sporicidal or tuberculocidal, organic matter interferes with their action, and they are readily neutralized by both soaps and anionic detergents. If they are used to disinfect any objects or surfaces that have been washed with soap or an anionic detergent and a residue remains, they are ineffective. Since it is recommended always to wash before attempting to disinfect, they have limited practical use in the hospital as disinfectants.

E. Alkylating Agents

Most alkylating agents are used in either the liquid or gaseous state. Their antimicrobial action is achieved through the alkylation of enzymes.

1. Formaldehyde

Sometimes used as a fumigant, formaldehyde is principally used as a fixative in solution as formalin for tissue specimens. It is highly irritable to live tissue, penetrates poorly, and leaves a residue.

2. Glutaraldehyde

a. Alkaline glutaraldehyde, buffered by a 0.3% NaCHO3 agent, is used in a 2% solution. It is bactericidal, tuberculocidal, and virucidal at room temperature in 10 minutes. It is sporicidal when applied for 10 hours. Once activated with the buffering solution, it is potent for 2 to 4 weeks, depending on the manufacturer. This varies slightly if equipment placed in it contains water, which dilutes the concentration of the compound. It is an irritant to the mucous membranes and eyes, so equipment that is sterilized or disinfected in it must be thoroughly rinsed before drying. Patients' tissues must not contact the residue. It is also a potent sensitizing agent. Once contact with skin causes sensitization, each additional contact increases sensitivity, which can lead to the development of extensive lesions. This fact reinforces the need for thorough rinsing of objects treated with alkaline glutaraldehyde. Rubber gloves must be used by personnel working with this solution. It cannot be used as an antiseptic. The health administration has set limits on exposure to glutaraldehyde. Glutaraldehyde is also used as a primary fixative agent for electron microscopy.

  b. Acid glutaraldehyde in a 2% solution is bactericidal and virucidal in 5 minutes, tuberculocidal in 20 minutes, and is sporicidal in 1 hour if the solution is heated to 60°C. Once in use it is potent for up to 30 days. Acid glutaraldehyde is not irritating to the eyes or mucous membranes, and gloves are not necessary when using it. It cannot be used as an antiseptic.

F. Ethylene Oxide Gas

Ethylene oxide (ETO) gas is a cyclic ether that forms explosive mixtures with air, and so is diluted with inert gases such as carbon dioxide, nitrogen, or halogenated hydrocarbons. The advantages of ETO are that it is penetrative and can sterilize without the use of high levels of heat or moisture though relative humidity levels of 30% to 60% are developed within the chamber, and this must be kept in mind when choosing objects for ETO sterilization. It is used for a wide range of articles that are affected by heat, including many items used in respiratory care. The disadvantages of ETO include the fact that it is explosive, is toxic if inhaled, and causes blisters on contact with the skin. It is also slow acting, compared to autoclaving, for example, and requires 4 hours of exposure at 50 to 56°C, or 6 to 12 hours at room temperature to produce sterility. A chemical indicator must be included with each batch of items that are processed. The method of microbial death is alkylation that is aided by the injected humidity level. The biological monitor used to check ETO sterilization contains *Bacillus subtilis var globigii.* Successful sterilization is dependent on several factors.

1. Items to be sterilized must be thoroughly cleaned and dried before processing.

2. Items must be wrapped in paper or muslin, or sealed in polyethylene bags, and placed in the sterilizer in a manner that the agent can reach all surfaces of the item.

3. Aeration in a mechanical aeration chamber for 8 hours at 60°C or 12 hours at 50°C is necessary for porous materials such as plastics to eliminate residue formation on items that will contact human tissue.

4. Because of the toxic nature of ETO, OSHA has recommended that minimal exposure to the gas by employees be accomplished by requiring adequate ventilation of the room in which ETO sterilization is performed, and that adequate aeration of processed items is performed in order to protect patients. Manufacturers' specifications for the use of ETO sterilizers and aerators must be strictly followed.

G. Silver Nitrate

Silver nitrate is classified as a heavy-metal disinfectant. In most states it is used by law in a 1% solution (Crede's method), instilled as a prophylactic measure into the eyes of newborn infants to prevent gonococcal ophthalmia neonatorum.

H. Chlorhexidine

Chlorhexidine is an antiseptic used in a 4% preparation for surgical scrubs, hand washing, and as a skin wound cleanser. It persists on the skin while not being significantly absorbed from the skin, is nonirritating, and is active against both gram-positive, and gram-negative organisms.

I. Other Antiseptics

Some other antiseptics commonly used in hospitals include povidone-iodine, benzalkonium chloride tincture or aqueous, and hydrogen peroxide.

SUGGESTED READING

Association for the Advancement of Medical Instrumentation. *Standards and Recommended Practices.* Vol 2: *Sterilization.* Arlington: Association for the Advancement of Medical Instrumentation, 1990.

Boyd, R. F. *Basic Medical Microbiology,* 5th ed. Boston: Little Brown, 1995.

Favero, M. S., and W. W. Bond. "Chemical Disinfection of Medical and Surgical Materials." In *Disinfection, Sterilization, and Preservation,* 4th ed. Edited by S. S. Block. Philadelphia: Lea and Febiger, 1991.

Occupational Safety and Health Administration. "Gluteraldehyde." *Federal Register* 54 (1989): 2464.

Rutala, W. A. "APIC Guidelines for Infection Control Practice: APIC Guidelines for Selection and Use of Disinfectants." *Amerian Journal of Infection Control* 18 (1990): 99–117.

Chapter 5

Aseptic Techniques

CHAPTER OBJECTIVES

Upon completion of this chapter, the reader will be able to

1. discuss the types of exposure that universal precautions are intended to prevent
2. compare and contrast the uses of the five types of gloves available to health care workers
3. define the concept of "sharps" and explain their proper handling
4. discuss the precautions necessary for personnel under each of the major categories of isolation
5. discuss the importance of hand washing, including the points at which it interrupts the transfer of microorganisms
6. list the circumstances in which hands should be washed
7. discuss the procedures in respiratory care that require following universal precautions

I. Isolation Precautions

Isolation precautions have been used in the United States since the 1700s when "fever hospitals" were opened during epidemics to prevent the spread of infection. They were usually closed after any particular epidemic was considered to be over. As early as 1877, publications recommended placing patients with communicable diseases in isolation huts, but this practice was not successful because patients with different communicable diseases were grouped together and aseptic techniques were not used. By 1889, however, hospitals began to separate patients according to particular diseases (cohorting), and aseptic techniques began to be observed. In 1910, isolation practices began to improve further, with the use of physical barriers between patients in isolation wards. The use of aseptic techniques included the use of gloves and gowns, disinfection of contaminated objects, and routine hand washing in those wards. As a group, these techniques came to be known as barrier nursing.

In the 1950s patients with infectious diseases began to be cared for in the general hospital setting, and in the 1960s tuberculosis hospitals across the nation were closed or converted to other uses. Patients with tuberculosis were then cared for in general hospitals in designated wards or rooms. In 1970 and 1975, the Centers for Disease Control (CDC) published a manual of isolation procedures that included isolation categories and techniques that were recommended for all hospitals. Despite the fact that most, if not all, hospitals implemented those recommendations, by the 1980s hospitals experienced endemic and epidemic nosocomial infection problems caused by multiple drug-resistant microorganisms, newly recognized syndromes, and infection problems in special-care units.

In 1993 the CDC published a new guideline that revised isolation categories and emphasized the necessity for physicians and nurses to individually evaluate patients' needs to be isolated. In 1985, largely as a result of the human immunodeficiency virus (HIV) epidemic, isolation practices in the United States were dramatically changed. A new concept in the approach to controlling transmissible blood-borne pathogens by applying an isolation category called "blood and body fluid precautions" was introduced.

Previous to 1985 that category was applied only to those patients who were known or suspected of having an infectious disease. As of 1985 it was recommended that blood and body fluid precautions apply to all patients. Thus, the term *universal* was adopted. Part of the new concept was the emphasis on the prevention of needle-stick injuries, and reemphasizing the use of barriers, including gloves and gowns as well as masks and eye coverings to prevent mucous membrane exposures.

Since that time, several reports from the CDC as well as proposals and regulations from the Occupational Safety and Health Administration (OSHA) and others have added to the concept of universal precautions.

II. Universal Blood and Body Fluid Precautions

Universal blood and body fluid precautions are intended to prevent parenteral, mucous membrane, and nonintact skin exposures in health care settings. While specific institutions can and should individualize policies and procedures to effect the concept of universal precautions based on factors such as the type of institution concerned or the population that the institution serves, in practice, the concept includes several factors and fundamental policies.

A. *Potentially* infectious materials include
- blood
- blood or serum-containing body fluids, secretions, or excretions
- any unfixed body tissue
- semen
- vaginal secretions
- cerebrospinal fluid
- synovial fluid
- plural fluid
- pericardial fluid
- amniotic fluid
- saliva
- excretions
- microbial cultures
- any other secretions

B. Procedures and policies recognized under the concept of universal blood and body fluid precautions include professional and patient protection.
  1. Hand washing before and after patient care immediately if contact made with potentially infectious material; and after removal of gloves or other personal protective equipment, e.g., masks or eye coverings.
  2. Contaminated gloves must be removed before handling a computer keyboard or phone. There are five general types of gloves.
     a. Surgeons' gloves, which are used for surgical procedures.
     b. Procedures gloves, which are used for procedures requiring a sterile and/or fitted glove (including bedside surgical procedures), and for procedures requiring manual dexterity.

    c. Exam gloves (vinyl or latex), which are used for short procedures that do not require significant dexterity.

    d. Dishwashing-type gloves, which are used for procedures in which resistance is important, e.g., cleaning of instruments or patient areas.

    e. Eudermic gloves, or other hypoallergenic gloves, which should be used by people who are sensitive to latex gloves.

3. Gowns or other protective clothing must be worn whenever soiling with potentially infectious materials may be reasonably anticipated. Clothing that has become soiled with potentially infectious material must be removed as soon as practical, and the area of skin that was soiled must be washed with soap and water.

4. Masks and eye protectors or face shields must be worn whenever splattering or aerosolization of potentially infectious material can be reasonably expected, e.g., during suctioning.

5. Sharps are medical articles that may cause punctures or cuts, and include needles, syringes, scalpel blades, suture needles, broken medical glassware, and disposable razors.

    a. Sharps must always be handled in a manner that prevents injury. They should be discarded immediately after use in an approved sharps container.

    b. Needles should not be recapped, bent, broken, or otherwise manipulated.

    c. Reaching into a sharps container should never be done *for any reason.*

    d. Sharps containers should be replaced as needed and never overfilled.

6. All penetrating injuries or possible exposure to potentially infectious material must be reported immediately by completing any needlestick/penetrating injuries and blood or secretions splash policy in force.

7. Used or soiled linen must be bagged in properly labeled bags according to institutional procedures, e.g., color of bags, and so forth. In particular, soiled linens should not be allowed to soak through their bags and leak fluids to the environment.

8. Contaminated trash must be placed in appropriate receptacles and disposed of according to local and state regulations.

9. Eating, drinking, applying cosmetics or lip balm, or handling contact lenses must not be done in areas where there is a likelihood of exposure to infectious materials.

10. Food and drink must not be kept or placed in refrigerators, freezers, shelves, cabinets, or on counters where potentially infectious materials are present or where they are stored.

11. All procedures involving potentially infectious materials must be performed in a manner that minimizes splattering or aerosolization.

12. Mouth pipetting (in a medical laboratory) of potentially infectious materials must never be done.

III. **Systems for Isolation Precautions**

There are two systems for isolation precautions recommended by the CDC.

A. Disease Specific Precautions

Disease specific precautions consider each case of infectious disease individually. Disease specific precautions are indicated for more than 150 diseases, syndromes, or conditions.

B. Category Specific Precautions

Category specific precautions group diseases for which similar isolation precautions are indicated. In practice, institutions, at the discretion of the infection committee, often combine the two systems but rely as the basis of their systems on the following six categories that are defined under the category specific precautions system.

1. Strict isolation is designed to prevent the transmission of highly contagious or virulent infections that can be spread by both air and contact.

   a. Diseases that require strict isolation include pharyngeal diphtheria, Lassa fever, and varicella or zoster in immunocompromised patients.

   b. In these instances a private room is indicated and the door should be kept closed. Patients infected with the same organism may share a room.

    c. Masks, gowns, and gloves are necessary for all persons entering the room, and hands must be washed after removal of gloves. Contaminated articles must be bagged and labeled before removal.

2. Contact isolation is designed to prevent the transmission of highly transmittable infections that do not warrant strict isolation. These infections are spread by close or direct contact.

    a. Diseases requiring contact isolation include acute respiratory infections in children, gonococcal conjunctivitis, herpes simplex infections, group A streptococcal infections, and multiple drug-resistant infections. Patients with major skin infections that are draining and that cannot be covered adequately with dressings also require contact isolation.

    b. In these instances a private room is indicated, but patients with infections with the same microorganism may share a room in some cases.

    c. Masks are necessary for those who come close to the patient, gowns are necessary if soiling is likely, gloves are indicated for touching infected material, and hands must be washed after removing gloves. Contaminated articles must be bagged and labeled before removal.

3. Respiratory isolation is designed to prevent the transmission of infectious diseases over short distances through the air (droplet transmission).

    a. Diseases requiring respiratory isolation include measles, *H. influenzae,* mumps, meningococcal disease, and pertussis.

    b. A private room is indicated in these instances also, but patients infected with the same organism may share a room, in some cases.

    c. Masks are necessary for those who come close to the patient, gowns and gloves are not indicated, and hands must be washed after touching the patient or after touching potentially contaminated articles. Contaminated articles must be bagged and labeled before removal.

4. Tuberculosis isolation is used for patients suspected or known to have infectious tuberculosis, including laryngeal tuberculosis. This category is referred to as Acid Fast Ba-

cillus (AFB) isolation on the isolation card placed on the door to the patient's room in order to protect patient's confidentiality.

a. It is recommended that patients with active infectious tuberculosis be placed in private rooms equipped with negative air-pressure systems that exhaust to the outside of the building.

b. Persons who enter the room should wear particulate respirators. Gowns are indicated if needed to prevent gross contamination of clothing, gloves are not indicated, and hands must be washed after touching the patient or potentially contaminated articles. Articles should be thoroughly cleaned before removal.

5. Enteric precautions is a category designed to prevent infections that are transmitted primarily by direct or indirect contact with fecal material.

a. Diseases requiring enteric precautions include diarrhea or gastroenteritis caused by amoebae, *Vibrio* genera, *E. coli, Salmonella, Shigella,* and *Giardia.*

b. A private room is not indicated unless the patient's hygiene is poor (does not wash after touching infective material, contaminates the environment, or shares contaminated materials).

c. Masks are not indicated, gowns are indicated if soiling is likely, gloves are indicated for touching infective material, and hands must be washed after removing gloves. Contaminated articles must be bagged and labeled before removal.

6. Drainage and secretion precautions are designed to prevent infections from being transmitted by direct or indirect contact with purulent material or drainage from an infected body site. A private room is not indicated, masks are not indicated, gowns are indicated if soiling is likely, and gloves are indicated for touching infected material. Hands must be washed after removing gloves. Contaminated articles must be bagged and labeled before removal.

C. Additional Concepts in Isolation Precautions

1. Resistant organism precautions is a category used in some institutions that applies to specific organisms as determined by each institution. Universal precautions are indi-

cated, and a private room may also be indicated. Two examples of organisms that may require the category of precaution are oxacillin-resistant *S. aureus* and chloramphenicol-resistant *H. influenzae*.

2. Protective isolation is a category of isolation precaution sometimes used in specific institutions to protect immunosuppressed and other individuals from infectious diseases. A private room is usually indicated. Persons with infection may not enter the room. Hands must be washed before touching the patient. Personnel assigned to the patient should not care for other infected patients. Other restrictions and the use of masks, gloves, or gowns are specified by physicians on an individual basis.

D. Body Substance Isolation

Body substance isolation is a system that has been proposed as an alternative to the systems recommended by the CDC. It focuses on the isolation of moist body substances through the use of barrier precautions for all patients and is diagnosis-driven regarding patients who have severe disease transmitted by the airborne route. Private rooms are required for patients with pulmonary tuberculosis and other diseases that have been grouped for strict isolation by the CDC. As with the CDC systems, hospitals have adopted some of the components of this system to fit their specific needs.

E. Special Areas

Some areas in hospitals, as a result of either the patient population that they serve or physical factors inherent in their design, present special problems in the control of infection. Special procedures have thus been developed through the infection committee. Included in these areas are operating rooms, recovery rooms, emergency rooms, outpatient surgical areas, and dental clinics. Infection control policies and procedures specified by the supervision in any special area must be followed by all personnel entering those areas. There are two areas of special interest to respiratory care practitioners.

1. Intensive-care units

Patients in intensive-care units (ICUs) of all types are at risk for contracting nosocomial infections, primarily because their normal host defenses are compromised by medical and surgical interventions such as vascular catheters, urinary catheters, endotracheal tubes, tracheostomy tubes, ulcer prophylaxis (which alters the flora of the stomach), and the fact that they often have underlying illnesses that impair their normal defenses. Additionally, they are grouped closely together with other patients who have a higher than usual chance of being infective.

a. Although it is recommended that all ICUs should have at least one class A isolation room (includes an anteroom for gowning and hand washing), many units do not. Even in the event that such a room is available, frequently more than one patient in a unit requires isolation precautions.

b. In practice, curtains and partitions as well as signs identifying the precautions required, e.g., gloves, are used to provide protection against transmission of microorganisms.

c. Individual institutions and intensive-care units develop procedures, basically barrier procedures, through infection control committees for specific situations.

2. Nurseries

Procedures for infection control in nurseries are specialized because of the nature of the patients (newborns acquire part of their microflora in nurseries) and the physical designs of nurseries.

a. Hand washing is thought to be the key in controlling infections in nurseries, and specialized hand washing procedures that include the use of an antimicrobial agent and a more thorough washing technique have been recommended (see IV, G).

b. Other recommended procedures include the following: personnel should wear scrub suits in the nursery and a gown when temporarily out of the nursery; all others entering the nursery should wear long-sleeved gowns over their clothing; a long-sleeved gown should be located at each bassinet for wear when the baby's body contacts personnel; gloves, masks, and caps should be used when judged appropriate.

c. Again, individual institutions and individual nurseries, e.g., premature, newborn, and so forth, set specific standards for infection control in those units. The CDC does recommend that forced air incubators not be substituted for private rooms in any nursery and that they not be relied on as a major means of preventing the transmission of infection.

IV. Techniques

A. Hand Washing

Hand washing is the single most important factor in preventing the spread of infection in the hospital. The use of antiseptic agents, antimicrobial drugs, and all other methods used to combat the spread of infection are ineffective when hospital employees do not wash their hands appropriately. Hand washing removes transient microbial contamination acquired from patients and contaminated objects. It therefore reduces the risk that the hands will serve as vectors for the transfer of microorganisms from one patient to another, from an object to a patient, from a patient to hospital personnel, and from one part of a patient's body to another (Figure 5–1).

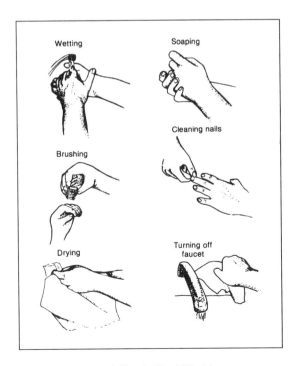

Figure 5–1 Standard 30-Second Simple Hand Washing.

1. Soaps and detergents aid in the hand washing procedure through their wetting, penetration, emulsification, and dispersive properties (see Chap. 4, IV, D, 1). Plain soap is usually preferred for routine hand washing.

2. Antimicrobial scrubs are agents that have an antimicrobial effect and should be used in hand washing before surgical procedures and in specified areas, e.g., nurseries, and under certain conditions, e.g., an outbreak of infection, as determined by specific institutions.

3. Hand brushes, scrub sponges, and manicure sticks aid in the removal of material from the fingernails and nail fold. Nails should be closely trimmed to facilitate effective handwashing.

B. When Hands Should Be Washed

Hands should be washed

- at the beginning and end of each shift
- after removal of gloves used in any contact with potentially infectious material
- after removal of gloves used in any isolation or precautions situation
- before and after any direct or indirect patient contact
- before and after performing any personal body functions for self or patient, including eating, removing contact lenses, using the bathroom, wiping or blowing nose, or combing hair
- before preparing or serving food or medications

C. Routine Hand Washing

Routine hand washing procedures differ in small respects from one institution to another, and employees must follow the recommended procedure used in the hospital in which they are employed. The following are presented as a "generic" routine hand washing procedure.

1. Turn on the faucet and adjust the flow and temperature of the water. Warm water is preferred, as it does not dry out the skin as much as hot water.

2. Wet hands to the wrists.

3. Apply soap to hands. If using solid soap, dig nails into the soap.

4. Rub hands together, using friction.

5. Wash between fingers and around nails.

6. Rinse hands thoroughly under running water.

7. Dry hands with a paper towel, moving from fingertips to wrists.
8. Turn off the faucet, using the towel for a hand-controlled faucet.
9. Discard the towel.

D. Lotion

Periodic application of an approved uncontaminated lotion to the hands is recommended because repeated hand washing, especially with antimicrobial agents, tends to irritate, dry, and crack the skin. Lotion contains ingredients that replace some of the natural skin oils that are removed by hand washing.

E. Exceptions

Under certain circumstances, for example, while transporting a patient in a vehicle, approved chemical solutions and cleansing pads may be used instead of washing. These circumstances are determined by the infection control committee.

F. Nonsurgical Scrubs

Nonsurgical scrub procedures are often used in areas or under circumstances in which a higher level of removal of microorganisms from the hands than is the result of the routine hand washing procedure is desired, e.g., an outbreak of infection in a small physical location. Often, the scrub must be performed for a specific amount of time, e.g., 15 seconds or 3 minutes depending on the circumstances, but a nonsurgical scrub procedure in a given situation usually involves the following eight steps.

1. Turn on the faucet and adjust the flow and temperature of the water.
2. Wet hands and arms to the elbows.
3. Apply antiseptic soap to the hands.
4. Holding hands upward (higher than elbows), wash, using friction; begin at fingertips and proceed up each arm to the elbow.
5. Rinse hands and arms thoroughly under running water.
6. Dry with two paper towels, using one for each hand and arm. Dry from fingers up each arm to elbow.
7. Turn off faucet, using the paper towels for a hand-controlled faucet.
8. Discard the towels.

G. Nursery
  A hand washing policy that has been recommended for nurseries includes a nonsurgical scrub and other features.
  1. On entering the nursery, personnel should remove jewelry from fingers and wrists and scrub hands and forearms to the elbows.
  2. An antiseptic agent such as an iodophor should be used.
  3. Thereafter, hands should be washed for 15 seconds before and after handling an infant or a potentially contaminated object. These washes may be done with plain soap.
  4. Hands should also be washed after touching one's hair, face, or body.
H. The 5-minute surgical scrub is necessary for surgical personnel and includes the use of a sponge impregnated with an antimicrobial preparation such as an iodophor, with sterile towels for drying. Between consecutive operations, the scrub must be performed again, but the duration may be as short as 2 minutes.

V. **Invasive Procedures in Respiratory Care**

Universal blood and body fluid procedures must be practiced in the performance of any invasive procedure.
A. Arterial Punctures
  Gloves must be worn while performing arterial punctures.
  1. Radial and brachial punctures require certain items and follow a certain procedure.
    a. Items needed: a micro sample kit or a sterile syringe, heparin, two needles, alcohol and/or Betadine swab, a sterile gauze pad, a sample bag with label, and a stopper or cork.
    b. Procedure
      (1) The first step in the procedure should be hand washing.
      (2) The Allen test must be performed in the case of a radial puncture.
      (3) The syringe must be prepared with heparin if it has not been heparinized by the manufacturer.
      (4) The puncture site is prepared with an alcohol or Betadine swab. Friction must be used in the application of the swab, using a circular motion, working from the potential puncture site outward.

(5) Palpate the artery, perform the puncture, and seal the syringe when the sample has been obtained.

(6) Apply pressure to the site with the gauze pad and place the syringe in ice.

(7) Continue to apply pressure to the site for 5 minutes by the clock.

2. There is some disagreement among physicians about the most desirable artery to be punctured in this procedure.

   a. Some physicians believe that the sequence of choice of sites should be the radial; the brachial; and only in certain circumstances and with physician consent, the femoral artery. They believe that the femoral puncture is the site of last resort because bleeding subsequent to the puncture is rapid and difficult to detect.

   b. Others believe that the brachial artery is the site of last resort because of the lack of collateral circulation to the areas served by that artery in the event that it collapses. These physicians prefer radial and femoral arteries as puncture sites.

   c. The procedure for puncture of the femoral artery is the same as for radial and brachial punctures, with the exception of the Allen test for radial punctures.

B. Cricothyroid Punctures

Transtracheal specimens are obtained by puncturing the cricothyroid membrane with a needle and aspirating a specimen.

1. Procedure

   a. A surgical scrub is recommended along with the use of sterile gloves, and the site should be prepared with antimicrobial solution.

   b. A local anesthetic is applied at the level of the cricothyroid membrane.

   c. The membrane is punctured with a needle.

   d. A No. 14 catheter is passed through the needle, and the specimen is collected.

2. Advantage

No oral flora is included in the sample.

3. Disadvantage

Invasive procedures are generally considered to be inherently less desirable than noninvasive procedures because of the possibility of infection. The complication rate for this procedure, however, is about 1%.

C. Bronchoscopic Samples

Bronchoscopic samples (sputum and tissue) are obtained through a bronchoscope and must be obtained under special conditions. The patient must be at least partially sedated, and a heart monitor should be used. An emergency drug tray should be immediately accessible. Oxygen must be administered to the patient during the procedure, and the patient should be monitored with a pulse oximeter.

1. Procedure
   a. First a topical anesthetic is applied in the nose, nasopharynx, and oropharynx down to the vocal cords.
   b. If the patient is connected to a ventilator, the F_{IO_2} should be increased during the procedure.
   c. Using aseptic technique, surgical scrub, and gloves, the scope is inserted.
   d. The secretions or tissue are visualized.
   e. The sample is collected. If a tissue sample is needed, the procedure should be performed with X-ray visualization of the forceps.
2. Advantages
   a. The sample is collected from a specific and known area of the lung.
   b. No oral flora is present.
3. Disadvantages
   a. A trained physician is needed to perform the procedure.
   b. The patient is discomforted by the procedure, especially if tissue is removed.
   c. If a rigid bronchoscope is employed, anesthesia is often necessary.
   d. Hypoxemia is a danger during the procedure.

VI. Noninvasive Procedures in Respiratory Care

A. Pharyngeal Culture

Pharyngeal cultures are considered to be noninvasive because the area to be sampled is easily reached with a swab through the mouth.

1. Bacterial
   a. Procedure
      (1) The sample is obtained by having the patient open his or her mouth. A cotton, dacron, or calcium algi-

nate swab is used to obtain the sample from the pharynx and tonsils.
   (2) The swab is then placed in culture media or transport media.
  b. Use
    Pharyngeal cultures are usually employed to detect diphtheria, pertussis, and gonococcus in children.
2. Viral
  a. Adults
   (1) The patient gargles with sterile broth containing 0.5% gelatin and expectorates into a collection cup.
   (2) The expectorant is immediately frozen.
  b. Children
    The pharynx is swabbed with the same mixture, and the specimen is placed in culture media or transport media.
B. Nasopharyngeal Culture
  1. The nasopharynx is swabbed with a cotton, dacron, or calcium alginate swab on a flexible wire.
  2. The swab is placed in culture media or transport media.
C. Other Sputum Samples
  1. Simple expectorated sputum
   a. Procedure
    (1) If possible, have the patient rinse his or her mouth and gargle with water prior to sputum collection.
    (2) The patient is asked to cough and expectorate into a sterile screw-cap cup, which is then labeled and sent to the laboratory.
    (3) Wash hands after handling the sputum cup.
   b. Advantage
    The procedure is accomplished with relative ease.
   c. Disadvantage
    Oral flora is present in the sputum.
  2. Induced sputum
   a. Procedure
    (1) If possible, have the patient brush the buccal mucosa, tongue, and gums with a wet toothbrush prior to the procedure.
    (2) The patient is asked to inhale a nebulized mist of 3% to 5% saline solution for a period of 5 to 30 minutes until a cough productive of sputum results.

The sputum is expectorated into a sterile screw-cap cup, which is labeled and sent to the laboratory.

(3) Wash hands after sputum is collected and remove equipment.

b. Advantage

The procedure is accomplished with relative ease compared with the invasive method when the patient has difficulty producing sputum without assistance.

c. Disadvantage

The sputum contains a considerable amount of oral flora.

3. Orotracheal and nasotracheal sputum specimens

This method is useful when a patient has difficulty producing or cannot produce a sputum sample, for example, in a comatose patient.

a. Procedure

(1) A suction catheter is used to remove a sputum sample from the patient's orotracheal or nasotracheal areas, and it is collected in an in-line sputum trap.

(2) The sputum trap is sealed, labeled, and sent to the laboratory.

(3) Wash hands after the procedure.

b. Advantage

Samples can be obtained from patients unable to produce sputum.

c. Disadvantage

As in the cases of simple and induced sputum samples, oral flora is present.

VII. Aseptic Nasotracheal Suctioning

Hands should be washed before and after each suction procedure when possible. Universal precautions must be followed.

A. Nasopharyngeal Suctioning

Nearly all hospitals today purchase prepackaged, sterilized suction kits to be used in these procedures.

1. Each kit should contain a lubricant or wetting reservoir (usually the kit package itself), a sterile glove, and at least one suction catheter. *These are disposable items, and no item in the kit should ever be used with more than one patient.*

2. The lubricants include normal sterile saline and a water-soluble lubricant. Petroleum-based lubricants should never be used.

3. If a patient is receiving oxygen through any type of appliance, whether nasal, cannula, mask, or ventilator, the patient must receive increased oxygen flow before, during, and after the procedure. Suction removes oxygen from the patient's lungs.

4. The glove is put on, and the catheter is connected to a vacuum source with the gloved hand holding the catheter. The vacuum is turned on.

5. Using the gloved hand, the catheter is lubricated before it is inserted into the patient.

B. Tracheal Suctioning

1. Without an endotracheal or tracheal tube, the procedure is the same as for nasopharyngeal suctioning but with three additional steps.

   a. Place patient in a high semi-Fowler's position.

   b. Measure from the anterior nares to the xiphoid process and hold the catheter at that length.

   c. Insert the catheter following its natural droop, and occlude the vent on the catheter to apply suction. Precaution: Apply suction for short periods, never more than 10 seconds at a time. Suctioning for longer periods can rapidly cause hypoxia and result in cardiac arrhythmias.

2. Through an endotracheal tube. Note the FiO_2 that the patient is receiving.

   a. Preoxygenate the patient by increasing FiO_2 to 1.0 (100%) for a period of 1 minute.

   b. Follow the same procedure described earlier. Precaution: Replace oxygen appliance intermittently at an FiO_2 higher than the patient was receiving prior to suction.

   c. After suctioning, reduce FiO_2 to normal level.

C. Disposal of Suction Kits

The kits, including all catheters, should be used and disposed of according to each hospital's infection control committee's and nursing service's guidelines.

D. Special Precautions

1. Routine removal of equipment

   a. All pneumatic and electric lines are disconnected.

  b. All disposable components should be disposed of in proper containers at the bedside.
  c. All permanent equipment is bagged and then returned to the cleaning area of the respiratory therapy department by as direct a route as possible according to departmental procedures.
  d. All equipment is then disassembled, washed, and disinfected and/or packaged for sterilization according to departmental procedures.
2. Removal of equipment from rooms of patients under isolation/precautions procedures
  a. Steps 1, a and b are followed.
  b. Equipment should be wiped down with a disinfectant solution and be placed in or covered by a labeled impervious plastic bag before removal from the room.
  c. Steps 1, c and d are then followed.

SUGGESTED READING

American Academy of Pediatrics and American College of Obstetricians and Gynecologists. *Guidelines for Perinatal Care.* Evanston: American Academy of Pediatrics, 1983.

American Thoracic Society, Centers for Disease Control. "Control of Tuberculosis." *American Review Respiratory Disease* 128 (1983): 336.

Bordley, J. *Two Centuries of American Medicine, 1776–1976.* Philadelphia: Saunders, 1976.

Centers for Disease Control. *Guidelines for the Prevention and Control of Nosocomial Infection: Guidelines for Handwashing and Hospital Environmental Control.* Atlanta: CDC, 1985.

Fahey, B. J., et al. "Frequency of Nonparenteral Occupational Exposures to Blood and Body Fluids Before and After Universal Precautions Training." *American Journal of Medicine* 90 (1991): 145.

Garner, J. S. "Universal Precautions and Isolation Systems." In *Hospital Infections,* 3d ed. Edited by J. V. Bennett and P. S. Brachman. Boston: Little, Brown, 1992.

Garner, J. S., and B. P. Simmons. "CDC Guideline for Isolation Precautions in Hospitals." *Infection Control* 4, Suppl. (1983): 245.

Goldman, D., et al. "Control of Hospital-Acquired Infections." In *Infectious Diseases in Medicine and Surgery.* Philadelphia: Saunders, 1992.

Goldman, D. A. "Epidemiology of Staphylococcus Aureus and Group A Streptococci." In *Hospital Infections,* 3d ed. Edited by J. V. Bennett and P. S. Brachman. Boston: Little, Brown, 1992.

Graham, M. "Frequency and Duration of Handwashing in an Intensive Care Unit." *American Journal of Infection Control* 18 (1990): 77.

Heinze, J. E. "Bar Soap and Liquid Soap (letter)." *Journal of American Medical Association* 251 (1984): 32222.

Hoeprich, P. D., M. C. Jordan, and A. R. Ronald. *Infectious Diseases,* 5th ed. Philadelphia: J. B. Lippincott, 1994.

Isenberg, H. D., ed. *Clinical Microbiology Procedures Handbook,* Suppl. 1. Washington, D.C.: American Society for Microbiology, 1994.

Jackson, M. M., and P. Lynch. "Isolation Practices: A Historical Perspective." *American Journal of Infection Control* 13 (1985): 21.

Klein, R. S. "Universal Precautions for Preventing Occupational Exposures to Human Immunodeficiency Virus Type 1." *American Journal of Medicine* 90 (1991): 141.

Nelson, J. D. "The Newborn Nursery." In *Hospital Infections,* 3d ed. Edited by J. V. Bennett and P. S. Brachman. Boston: Little, Brown, 1992.

Nichols, R. L. "The Operating Room." In *Hospital Infections,* 3d ed. Edited by J. V. Bennett and P. S. Brachman. Boston: Little, Brown, 1992.

Occupational Safety and Health Administration. "Occupational Exposure to Bloodborne Pathogens: Final Rule." *Federal Register* 56 (6 December 1991): 64004–82.

Pittet, D., L. A. Herwaldt, and R. M. Massanari. "The Intensive Care Unit." In *Hospital Infections,* 3d ed. Edited by J. V. Bennett and P. S. Brachman. Boston: Little, Brown, 1992.

Wenzel, R. P., and M. A. Pfaller. Handwashing: Efficacy Versus Acceptance: A Brief Essay. *Journal of Hospital Infection* 18, Suppl. B (1991): 65.

Williams, W. W. "CDC Guideline for Infection Control in Hospital Personnel." *Infection Control* 4, Suppl. (1983): 326.

Wong, E. S., et al. "Are Universal Precautions Effective in Reducing the Number of Occupational Exposures among Health Care Workers?" *Journal of American Medical Association* 265 (1991): 1123.

Chapter 6

Preparation of Equipment for Sterilization and Disinfection

CHAPTER OBJECTIVES

Upon completion of this chapter, the reader will be able to

1. discuss the basic design principles of an area for processing respiratory care equipment
2. explain the importance of the proper labeling of packages containing sterilized equipment
3. discuss the factors involved in choosing reusable or disposable materials in respiratory care and why a mixed materials system is often chosen
4. compare and contrast the three categories of items in Spaulding's classification system

After equipment has been used in patient care areas, it must be returned to the designated cleaning area for processing. Effective processing of equipment provides an aseptic barrier between patient uses and is dependent on the design of the cleaning area among other factors.

I. **The Cleaning Area** (Figures 6–1 and 6–2)

    A. Design

        Design of the cleaning area is based on a few simple principles.

        1. Areas in which equipment is cleaned must be physically separated from areas in which ready-to-use equipment is stored. In Figure 6–1, the barrier is a 7-foot-high partition with the upper 3-foot area being made of Plexiglas so that

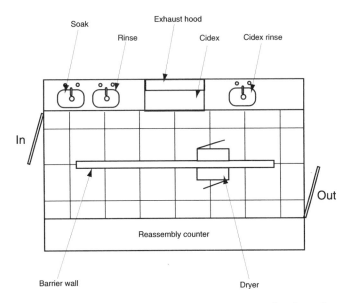

Figure 6–1 Design for a Respiratory Care Equipment Processing Area. *Source:* Original design by David M. Ayars, III, CRTT, Director of Cardiopulmonary Services, Memorial Hospital of Salem County, Salem, New Jersey.

personnel on each side are able to see what those on the other side are doing. An equipment drier that has doors on both sides so that equipment that has been treated and dried may be passed through from the contaminated side to the processed side has been incorporated. This design is close to ideal for an area of limited size.

2. An exhaust hood should be located in the area where glutaraldehyde is used in order to protect the staff from fumes.

3. A specific pathway for equipment from patient care areas should be established through the cleaning area.

4. Ready-to-use equipment should never be moved through the cleaning area. The entrance used to bring equipment into the cleaning area should never be used to exit ready-to-use equipment.

5. An assembly and testing area should be located between the cleaning and ready-to-use areas.

6. The area used for reports by the staff should be physically separate from the cleaning assembly and ready-to-use areas.

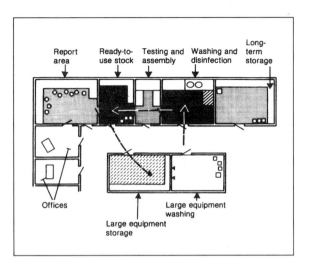

Figure 6–2 Alternative Floor Plan, with Work Flow Indicated.

B. Work Flow

The department should be designed in such a manner that the physical facilities are organized in accordance with the equipment processing procedures. This aids in ensuring that disinfection and sterilization will be properly accomplished, and it makes the process more efficient.

1. The facilities should be arranged so there is a doorway through which unprocessed equipment enters.
2. There is a contaminated- or dirty-equipment area.
3. The washing area should have a double, stainless steel sink for washing and rinsing equipment by hand. Large equipment may also be wiped down in this area. A hand washing sink should be available for use after handling contaminated equipment.
4. The sterilization and disinfection area is the location of chemical solutions, ultrasonic sterilizers, pasteurizing equipment, and small autoclave.
5. A wrapping area for items to be autoclaved or gas sterilized should be located across from the sterilization and disinfection area.
6. Drying should be performed on the same side of the room but just past the sterilization and disinfection area.

7. The assembly and testing area should be located so that sterilized and disinfected equipment can pass directly into it.

8. The staff report area and supervisor offices should be located so that access to them is possible without one's having to pass through the contaminated, washing, sterilization and disinfection, wrapping, or drying areas. It is not necessary for the report and office areas to be accessible without passing through the assembly and testing area.

C. Washing

Every piece of equipment used in a patient care area should be washed with soap and water and treated with a suitable disinfectant before it is used in another patient's room. This helps prevent any equipment from acting as a vector in the hospital. Since there is no visible means to determine if a given item has been contaminated in use, all equipment should be given this minimum processing.

1. Hand washing

a. Equipment composed of more than one piece should be disassembled into as many component parts as recommended by the manufacturer.

b. Equipment with organic contaminants such as blood or mucous should be soaked in hot water with an alkaline soap and scrubbed with a brush. It then must be rinsed with water before any further processing.

2. Mechanical washing

If an automatic washing machine such as an ultrasonic washer is available, the process is a two-step one.

a. Equipment should be disassembled into as many component parts as recommended by the manufacturer.

b. Equipment is placed in the washer. The washer is activated and the equipment is removed when the washing cycle is completed.

D. Wrapping

There are two categories of equipment that are wrapped in the cleaning area (Figure 6–3).

1. First are the items that have been washed and will be autoclaved or gas sterilized in another department. The wrapping area should be stocked with wrapping materials and indicator tape of the kinds standard for the hospital. Materials used for wrapping items to be autoclaved include pa-

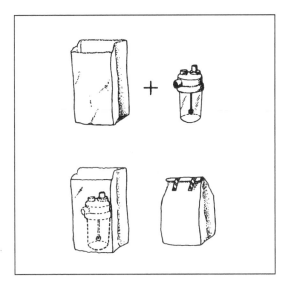

Figure 6–3 Packaging a Nebulizer for Steam Autoclaving. The top of the bag is folded over tightly several times and sealed with indicator tape.

per bags, linen, and muslin. Materials used for wrapping items to be sterilized with ethylene oxide (ETO) gas are wrapping paper, cloth, muslin, polyethylene, and nylon film. Examples of objects in this category are nebulizers, spirometers, and bacterial filters.

2. Second are the items that have been sterilized or disinfected in the respiratory-therapy department. Usually, at least some of the equipment used by respiratory-care practitioners is processed entirely in the department. Examples are large-bore ventilator tubing, manifolds, and manual resuscitators. After such items are sterilized or disinfected, dried, and assembled, they must be wrapped to keep them as clean as possible before their next use. Only items that do not need to be sterile when placed in patient use may be processed in the department. Wrapping items after sterilization and disinfection assures that such items are not sterile.

E. Sterilization and disinfection

The methods used to accomplish sterilization and disinfection in the respiratory-therapy department vary.

1. Sterilization

   Treating an item so that it is ready for use in a sealed sterile package is probably only possible if a small gas sterilizer or small autoclave is available within the department.

2. Disinfection

   Many of the methods utilized in the respiratory-therapy department do sterilize the items treated at some point. However, rinsing or packaging the items subsequent to the sterilization renders them not sterile but clean. That is, the infectious microorganisms have been killed, but other nonpathogenic microorganisms are present on the items. The usual methods of disinfection in a respiratory-therapy department are through the use of chemicals, pasteurization, and ultrasound.

   a. Chemical disinfection takes place when a chemical agent is used to disinfect equipment, and six precautions must be taken.

      (1) There must be proper air exchange in the room where equipment is processed in accordance with Occupational Safety and Health Administration (OSHA) standards.

      (2) Equipment that has been washed must be drained prior to immersion in the chemical agent. Residual water on equipment after washing and rinsing dilutes the chemical agent, thus rendering it less potent. Therefore, many departments test these agents for potency once a week.

      (3) Strict attention must be paid to the active life of the chemical agent. The date of activation of the agent should be clearly displayed on the container of the solution. The chemical agent must be disposed of after passing the period of time specified by the manufacturer. If this is not done, the solution loses its potency and microorganisms may survive being immersed.

      (4) Any item processed with a chemical agent must be immersed for the amount of time specified by the manufacturer or microbial killing will be incomplete.

      (5) All items disinfected in a chemical agent must be thoroughly rinsed with water before drying and as-

sembly. The residues of chemical agents are irritating to tissue.

    (6) All items processed in a chemical agent should then be dried, reassembled, and wrapped before storage. The date of disinfection must be noted on the package.

  b. Pasteurization takes place when a pasteurization machine (Figure 6–4) is used for equipment disinfection. All items should be dried, reassembled, and packaged before storage. The date of pasteurization must be noted on the package.

  c. Ultrasonic disinfection takes place when equipment is processed in an ultrasonic sterilizer. Equipment should be rinsed with water, dried, reassembled, and packaged. The package must be dated.

F. Labeling

Anything that is sterilized or disinfected must be labeled with the date on which that item is processed along with the method used. This is absolutely necessary because the time in which the item is suitable for use after processing varies with the process. If the packaging material is anything other than

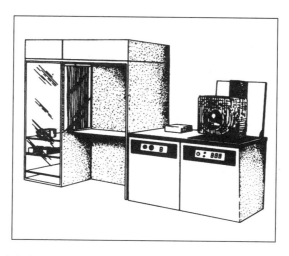

Figure 6–4 A Complete Pasteurizing System Including Washer, Pasteurizer, Assembly Hood, and Forced Air Drier.

clear plastic, it must also be labeled with the contents. Otherwise, packages will be opened needlessly.

1. Items that were autoclaved are suitable for use if the package is intact for 30 days.

2. Items sterilized by gas in an intact package are suitable for use for a period of 1 year.

3. Items processed chemically, those pasteurized, and those processed in an ultrasonic sterilizer in an intact package are suitable for use for 30 days after processing.

G. Rotation of Materials

Packaged disinfected items must be rotated in storage so that those least recently used are put into circulation in the hospital. This helps prevent expiration dates from passing while items are in storage. If this does occur, the item must be repackaged and reprocessed; they may not be used (Figure 6–5).

H. Ready-To-Use Materials

Materials to be used in patient care areas, including permanent large equipment and disposable supplies, must not be stored in the cleaning area. They must be stored in such a manner that the integrity of their packaging is not endangered and where they will not get wet. Any package that becomes wet must be reprocessed and repackaged. Materials should be stored in a logically convenient manner. For example,

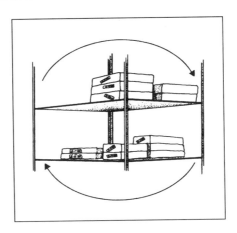

Figure 6–5 Sterile Supplies Must Be Rotated Back to Front as They Are Used.

nebulizers, oxygen tubing, and various oxygen appliances should be stored so that they all can be easily reached without a person taking a step. This is especially true for any emergency supplies, such as endotracheal tubes and stylettes. Long-term storage and bulk storage of supplies should be in a clean, dry area close to the department.

II. Selecting a Materials Supply System

Respiratory-therapy materials (supplies that are not capital items) are either disposable (single-patient use) or reusable and must be disinfected between uses. In purchasing these materials, the chief therapist can make one of three choices.

A. All Reusable Materials

Reusable materials such as humidifiers, nebulizers, and intermittent positive-pressure circuits are expensive when compared to their disposable equivalents (Figure 6–6). However, their initial cost must be spread out according to the number of times that they can be used. They are normally of sturdier construction than disposable units used for the same purpose. Each patient use of a reusable item is comparatively inexpensive. But the cost of labor to process reusables as well as the

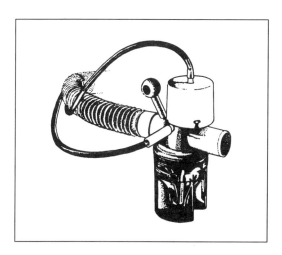

Figure 6–6 Example of a Disposable IPPB Circuit That Should Not Be Reused.

cost of purchasing and maintaining parts for them must be
added to the initial cost (purchase price).

B. All Disposable Materials

Disposable materials have the advantage that they are taken
fresh from their package for each new patient and eliminate
the problem of cross-contamination with their use, assuming
that they are used properly, that is, for one patient only. They
are generally not as sturdy as reusable materials, and if they
are broken or are malfunctioning, they cannot be repaired.
They are expensive to use on a single patient compared to permanent materials, especially if they are not purchased in bulk.
They also present a danger in that an uninformed or overly
cost-conscious therapist may attempt to disinfect and reuse
them. Disposables are not constructed of materials suitable for
disinfection and are not to be used by more than one patient.

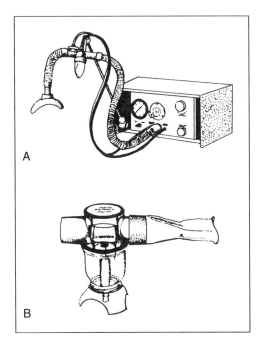

Figure 6–7 A. Example of a Standard IPPB Unit with Permanent Tubing-Mani-
fold Assembly. B. Disposable Manifold and Mouthpiece.

C. A Mixed Materials System

Most hospitals find a system of purchasing both reusable and disposable materials to be to their advantage (Figure 6–7). An all-reusable system is really only theoretic because items like oxygen tubing are not available in a reusable form. An entirely disposable system is simply too expensive for most hospitals. A system that utilizes reusable items where durability is important and disposables when rapid turnaround time is necessary is probably the most practical one. Whenever possible, disposable materials should be used whenever a patient is placed in isolation.

III. Mixed Levels of Asepsis

Items used in patient care vary in the level of necessary asepsis, in the necessary processing, according to their use, and as a result of other factors. The level of necessary asepsis must be determined for everything used in patient care areas—from bed linen to tracheostomy tubes. The responsibility for determining the level of necessary asepsis for any given item falls on several members of hospital personnel, primarily the infection control committee members and the medical director of each specific department. The decisions involving the procedures necessary for accomplishing the appropriate levels of asepsis are the responsibility of the committee medical directors, the infection control nurse, the head of the central supply department, and other department heads.

A. The most common approach to this problem is to utilize some version of Spaulding's classification system, which categorizes items into three groups based on their use in patient care.

1. Critical items are those that enter tissue or vascular space and require sterilization. Examples include arthroscopes, laparoscopes, and cardiac catheters.

2. Semicritical items are those that contact intact mucous membranes or nonintact skin, and require high-level disinfection. Some semicritical items such as fiber-optic bronchoscopes should ideally be sterilized but as a result of their construction are usually only disinfected.

3. Noncritical items are those that contact intact skin and require intermediate- or low-level disinfection. Examples include bedpans, urinals, and crutches.

B. In practice, decisions about how specific items will be processed involve several factors.

1. If an object is to be used for invasive procedures, for example, it must arrive at the procedure location sterile and in a protective package, that item must have been either autoclaved, gas sterilized, or irradiated while in a sealed package. However, many items such as ventilator tubing do not need to be sterile. In fact, these items, because of handling when they are put into use, cannot be sterile. They must be disinfected after use and uncontaminated when reused.

2. The physical composition of the item to be processed must be considered. Many objects cannot be autoclaved because the process will either damage or destroy them, for example, delicate surgical instruments and most products made of plastics. Other items cannot be processed with ETO because they will combine chemically with the gas and a toxic residue will result.

3. The amount of time required to perform sterilization or disinfection, drying, assembly, and packaging of items is also a factor in the choice of method of processing. For example, reusable humidifiers can well withstand gas sterilization. However, since that process requires aeration time after sterilization, gas sterilization may be impractical because it requires the purchase of a large number of humidifiers so that a sufficient number are available while others are being used. In this case, autoclaving would be the procedure of choice because it provides the same level of asepsis (sterile in package) but does not require a lengthy aeration time.

4. The nature of the contaminating organism is a consideration in the processing of objects in two ways.

   a. For immunosuppressed patients or others at special risk of becoming infected, such as burn patients, careful processing of items to be used in the patient's care must be observed. Such patients can be overwhelmed by infection with a microorganism that would not harm patients with intact immune systems. Therefore, the level of asepsis for materials to be used in their treatment should be as high as possible. Any sterile object that can reach the immunosuppressed patient should arrive sterile. The use of disposable products is highly desirable.

b. Objects that are returned from isolation must be handled differently from those routinely processed. An example is the object used by a patient with active tuberculosis. This must be disinfected prior to washing for the protection of the cleaning personnel (see Chap. 5).

IV. Procedures Manuals

Timely procedures manuals for the processing of equipment and aseptic standards for patient care supplies must be available to the respiratory staff at all times. There is no room for guesswork on the staff's part regarding either the method of decontamination or the level of asepsis necessary for any item maintained by the department.

A. A procedures manual should be updated at least annually by supervisors in consultation with the infection control nurse, medical director, staff, and the head of central supply.

B. Instructions regarding both processing and in-use procedures should be written for every item and every procedure for which the department is responsible.

C. Procedures for specific pieces of equipment and in-use procedures should be indexed and easily found in the manual.

D. Procedures manuals should be kept in an easily accessible place for staff members' use. Procedures manuals are of no use if they are locked in a supervisor's office. They are written to be used, not displayed to accreditation teams. They are tools that enable staff members to perform their jobs properly and minimize the possibility of spreading nosocomial infections.

SUGGESTED READING

Association for the Advancement of Medical Instrumentation. *Standards and Recommended Practices.* Vol 2: *Sterilization.* Arlington: Association for the Advancement of Medical Instrumentation, 1990.

Emergency Care Research Institute. "Ethylene Oxide: Hazards and Safe Use." *Technol. Respir. Therapy* 9, 12 (1989): 1–4.

Favero, M. S., and W. W. Bond. "Chemical Disinfection of Medical and Surgical Materials." In *Disinfection, Sterilization, and Preservation,* 4th ed. Edited by S. S. Block. Philadelphia: Lea and Febiger, 1991.

Haney, P. E., B. A. Raymond, and L. C. Lewis. "Ethylene Oxide. An Occupational Health Hazard for Hospital Workers." *AORN Journal* 51, 2 (1990): 480–1, 485–6.

Rahame, F. S. "The Inanimate Environment." In *Hospital Infections,* 3d ed. Edited by J. V. Bennett and P. S. Brachman. Boston: Little, Brown, 1992.

Rutala, W. A. "APIC Guidelines for Infection Control Practice: APIC Guidelines for Selection and Use of Disinfectants." *American Journal of Infection Control* 18 (1990): 99–117.

Scanlan, C. L., and H. St. Hill. "Principles of Infection Control." In *Eagan's Fundamentals of Respiratory Care,* 6th ed. Edited by C. L. Scanlan, C. B. Spearman, and R. L. Sheldon. St. Louis: 1995.

Spaulding, E. H. "Chemical Disinfection and Antisepsis in the Hospital." *Journal of Hospital Residency* 9 (1972): 7–31.

Chapter 7

Sterilization and Disinfection of Equipment

CHAPTER OBJECTIVES

Upon completion of this chapter, the reader will be able to

1. explain the importance of the proper processing of nebulizers
2. describe the reasons why fiber-optic bronchoscopes are usually hand processed
3. compare and contrast the uses of tap water and sterile water in respiratory care
4. compare and contrast the types of filters used in respiratory care

As a result of the nature of the materials used in the manufacture of respiratory therapy equipment and supplies and the variety of their applications, no single sterilization or disinfection process can be recommended. The methods of sterilization and disinfection most often used in respiratory therapy are autoclaving, sterilization with ethylene oxide (ETO) gas, chemical sterilization or disinfection, and pasteurization. The method chosen is most often selected on the basis of the composition of the item to be treated.

I. Sterilization and Disinfection between Patient Uses

A. Humidifiers

At least two types of humidifiers and often more are used for different purposes in any given hospital. It has generally been suggested that since humidifiers do not generate water droplets as do nebulizers, they need not be subjected to the more rigorous sterilization or disinfection processes recommended for nebulizers (autoclaving, ETO sterilization). However, the processing of humidifiers should be as rigorous as possible.

Humidifiers used for gas therapy should be subjected to the same processes as are nebulizers. Permanent humidifiers are constructed of the same materials as permanent nebulizers, so there is no reason not to process them along with nebulizers. Disposable humidifiers should not be reused.

B. Nebulizers

The construction of nebulizers varies greatly, and this dictates the use of different methods of sterilization or disinfection.

1. Reusable nebulizers include pneumatic nebulizers, which can be disinfected in chemical sterilizing agents or through pasteurization, but since they produce water particles and introduce them into the respiratory system, it is safest to wash, wrap, and sterilize them through autoclaving or ETO sterilization. Care must be taken not to attach the nebulizer jar tightly to the top prior to wrapping so as to ensure exposure of all areas to the sterilizing agent. Tightly screwed-on jar tops can bind to the washer as a result of the heat in the autoclave. Nebulizers should not be removed from their wrapping material until they are to be used. The outside of the wrapping material (usually paper bags) should be marked with the word *nebulizer,* the date of processing, and the initials of the person who prepared the nebulizer for sterilization. Disposable nebulizers should never be reused.

2. Croupettes and croup tents incorporate nebulizers as an integral part of the croupette body. The nebulizer must be disassembled as far as possible, and those parts must be washed and treated with a chemical agent, rinsed, and dried. The body of the device must be wiped down with soapy water and a chemical agent, rinsed, and dried. Reusable canopies are processed in the same manner. The croupette body, canopy, and nebulizer parts must be dried before reassembly. Whenever practical, disposable canopies should be used.

3. Ultrasonic nebulizers are composed of two basic units.

a. The ultrasound generator and fan unit must be wiped down with soapy water and a chemical disinfectant. Reusable filters must be removed, washed, chemically treated, rinsed with water, and dried. Disposable filters are discarded. If the nebulizer is operated from a portable stand, the stand and wheels should be wiped down with soapy water and a chemical agent.

    b. Disposable solution cups should not be reused; they should be discarded. Reusable solution cups should be treated with a chemical agent, rinsed, and dried. If any other form of disinfection or sterilization is considered, refer to the manufacturer's instructions. Waterfed systems for ultrasonic nebulizers must be selected and used with care because in the case of contamination of the system, large amounts of contaminated water will be directed toward the patient's respiratory system.

C. Portable Gas-Generating Delivery Systems

    1. Air compressors should be wiped down with soapy water and detergent. Any filters (they are all reusable) must be washed and dried. Condensation pans must be emptied and wiped down with soapy water.

    2. Flow meters and regulators. Gas-mixing devices should be wiped down with soapy water and a chemical agent. They must never be immersed in any solution, and contamination with any oily substance must be avoided. If such contamination does occur, the item must be scrupulously cleaned before reuse. Contact between oxygen and oily substances creates heat and a fire may result. Acetone can be used to remove oil from devices. Acetone is explosive and highly volatile, so it must be stored in a fireproof container and used in a ventilated area. If acetone is to be used in the department, the hospital laboratory should be contacted for specific instructions for its safe use.

    3. Cylinder transport carts should be periodically wiped down with soapy water and a chemical agent. The wheels should not be neglected in this process.

D. Heating Devices

    Devices that are used to heat water in humidifiers or nebulizers must be processed with care because they are electric appliances.

    1. Surfaces that contact the interior of the water reservoir should be wiped down with soapy water and a chemical agent for the proper length of time, rinsed, and dried before use.

2. Other surfaces such as the electric cord and plug must never be immersed and should be wiped down carefully with a chemical agent so that fluids do not enter any of the electric components.

3. Reservoirs of heated humidifiers may be processed by pasteurization, immersion in a chemical agent, autoclaving, or treatment with ETO, although treatment with ETO is not usually cost-effective for these items.

E. Intermittent Positive-Pressure Breathing (IPPB) Devices

The processing of IPPB devices varies somewhat with the manufacturer, and specific information should be requested. There are, however, some basic procedures that are recommended.

1. The entire surface of the device, including wheels, should be wiped down with soapy water and a chemical agent. Removable filters should be periodically washed, treated with a chemical agent, rinsed, and thoroughly dried. Processing includes any electric or pneumatic lines.

2. Accessible valve mechanisms should be wiped with soapy water, treated with a chemical agent, and rinsed.

3. If IPPB therapy is to be given without the use of a bacterial filter in line, a practice that the author condemns, most IPPB devices can be treated with ETO gas in a chamber equipped for such devices. Manufacturers' instructions for this procedure must be solicited, and special arrangements must be made with the person responsible for the use of the ETO chamber. A lengthy aeration period is required for IPPB devices treated with ETO.

F. Portable Spirometry Devices

1. Reusable portable spirometry devices are fragile instruments, and great care must be exercised in their processing.

a. These devices must never be immersed in any solution, but they may be wiped down with aqueous alcohol. Contamination with organic materials is a rare event for these devices because there is no reason for them to be placed in contact with surfaces or patients. Moving parts must not be touched or damage will result.

b. Treatment with ETO gas is the process of choice for these instruments because it is thorough and no manipulation of moving parts is necessary. The relative humidity of an ETO chamber is not high enough to damage the instruments.

   c. Portable spirometry devices must be carefully packaged prior to ETO processing and carefully handled during the loading and unloading of the chamber in order to avoid damage.

  2. Disposable spirometry devices should be discarded when their use is discontinued. Attempts at sterilizing or disinfecting these devices should not be made because the processes are incompatible with their construction and composition.

G. Manual Resuscitators

Resuscitators must be disassembled as completely as possible, washed, sterilized or disinfected, rinsed, and dried after each use. Since the materials and designs of manual resuscitators vary greatly, specific instructions must be obtained from manufacturers. Although obtaining this information is recommended prior to establishing processing procedures for all equipment, it is essential in the case of manual resuscitators because they are used in life-threatening situations. Mechanical failure in use as a result of inappropriate sterilization or disinfection must be avoided at all costs. Further, the use of a manual resuscitator with more than one patient without proper processing exposes such patients to another potentially fatal situation—a nosocomial pulmonary infection.

H. Electrically Powered Volume Ventilators

Of all devices used in respiratory care, the electrically powered volume ventilator is the most complex device to process after patient use.

  1. The filters for both the cooling fan and compressor intake must be washed in soapy water and dried before they are replaced.

  2. The entire ventilator must be wiped down with soapy water and a chemical agent, including the electric and pneumatic lines. Any shelves that are integral to the ventilator should be cleared of any items, such as tubing adapters, and wiped down with soapy water and a chemical agent. All items removed from the ventilator should be appropriately processed or discarded.

       3. Periodically the copper bead filter located at the oxygen and/or compressed air inlets should be removed and washed in soapy water, then rinsed and dried.

I. Fiber-optic Bronchoscopes

These extremely delicate and very expensive instruments must be sterilized or disinfected after each patient use. The use of chemical agents is the preferred method to date.

       1. The instrument must first be tested for leaks, then washed with warm soapy water, utilizing the cleaning brush provided by the manufacturer. Brushes obtained from sources other than the manufacturer must not be used; they could seriously damage the instrument. Soapy water is used to wipe down the exterior and is passed through it with the use of a large syringe. The bronchoscope is then rinsed in a similar manner.

       2. Sterilization or disinfection is accomplished by suspending the instrument in a tall beaker containing a chemical agent. A small syringe is used to draw the agent up the full length of the inner channel and remains attached for the period of time recommended by the instrument's manufacturer.

       3. It is then thoroughly rinsed, preferably with sterile water and a sterile syringe, air dried with care, and packaged. It is particularly important that this instrument be well rinsed and dried because its potential for causing irritation to lung tissue, should residue of the chemical agent remain, is enormous.

       4. Because the instrument is so fragile and because of its potential role in spreading disease as a nondisposable invasive instrument, only specially trained individuals should have access to the fiber-optic bronchoscope.

J. Endotracheal Tubes

Tracheal intubation is an invasive procedure; therefore, the tubes inserted should have as high a level of asepsis as possible. Because respiratory therapists usually perform tracheal intubation under life-threatening conditions, it is generally safest to use disposable endotracheal tubes that are sterile and prepackaged. The tubes should not be removed from their packages until the last feasible moment prior to use. Whenever possible, they should be removed from the package, using aseptic procedure, and inserted immediately. They should not be placed on the patient's bed or stretcher before they are inserted. Often the physical difficulties involved in emergency intubation, such as regurgitation or physical damage to the upper airway, make any attempt at asepsis futile, but aseptic technique should be followed as closely as possible. Any contamination introduced to the patient's lungs during the procedure will cause serious problems later.

II. Procedures for Equipment in Use

Given the most careful processing of equipment prior to use, a number of precautions are necessary after equipment is placed in use at the bedside.

A. Water

Water is one of the most commonly used substances in respiratory care. It is available in various stages of asepsis and containers.

1. Tap water is used in respiratory therapy for washing and rinsing equipment. The advantages of tap water are its ready availability and low cost. Its disadvantages are that it contains many impurities that tend to adhere to and corrode equipment and that it contains hospital flora. Cultures of pathogenic microbes are easily obtained from virtually any faucet or sink in a hospital. Therefore, tap water must never be used in any nebulizer or in a humidifier that is used for the administration of gas therapy.

2. Sterile bottled water is the type of water used for the bulk of patient care procedures. It may be either distilled or not distilled. It is used to irrigate wounds, soak dressings, lubricate catheters, and rinse sterilized equipment while maintaining sterility, and if distilled, it is used in humidifiers and nebulizers both as a wetting agent and as a carrier for medications. Its advantages are that it contains neither impurities, which harm equipment, nor normal hospital flora, though some highly resistant hospital-based pathogens have been isolated from so-called sterile distilled water. The disadvantages of sterile distilled water are that it is comparatively expensive, and it may contain preservatives and antipyrogens that can be irritating to respiratory mucosa. The use of sterile water for routine washing and rinsing of equipment is prohibitively expensive as well as impractical. When a bottle of sterile water is opened, it must be marked with the date and time of opening. All opened,

undated bottles must be discarded. Since opened bottles of any type of water can be major sources of agents that cause nosocomial infection, and since respiratory therapists constitute a majority of the people using sterile water in the hospital, the dating of bottles should be stressed in all procedures that require the use of sterile water.

B. Filters

Filtration of medical gases and liquids is necessary in several stages prior to the administration of therapy.

1. Gross filters are used for trapping the visible debris and particles that are classified as gross. The brass bead filters located at the compressed gas inlets of devices such as ventilators as well as the air filters on compressors and equipment driers are gross filters. They trap dirt, dust, and other soil that is visible to the eye and must be periodically cleaned to ensure the proper functioning of the equipment they protect. Other gross filters are the various plastic meshes and synthetic sponges used in nebulizers for essentially the same purpose. Gross filters are usually not disposable.

2. Bacterial filters are used to provide bacteria-free therapeutic gases to patients. They are very thin, porous sheets of cellulose esters and other materials that are encased in variously shaped canisters. These filters, essential to safe respiratory therapy, may be either single use (disposable) or reusable. Reusable filters must be autoclaved after every use. Some must not be immersed in any solution and must be discarded if immersion occurs. Reusable filters must be periodically tested according to manufacturers' specifications since they lose effectiveness with use. When first put into use, they must be dated with ink that cannot be removed or engraved with the date. There are two types of bacterial filters.

a. Mainstream filters are used in the mainstream flow circuit of ventilators and IPPB devices. These devices should not be used without mainstream filters, especially when gas is delivered through an endotracheal or tracheal tube.

b. Sidestream filters are fitted in the nebulizer lines on ventilators and IPPB devices. Their use is recommended, but their importance is less than the mainstream filters' importance because they often filter only oxygen on IPPB devices, and nebulizers on ventilators are used infrequently. Bacterial filters that can be used with nebulizers to filter entrained hospital air are sorely needed but to date have not been designed.

c. Viral filters are similar in construction to bacterial filters, but they also remove viruses from gases. They are more expensive than bacterial filters and to date have gained only limited acceptance, since viral infection from therapeutic gases is not considered to be a major problem, at least in comparison to bacterial infection.

d. Sophisticated filtrating devices are available for use with large compressors used to provide air for medical uses. Such compressed-air systems can remove oil and particles as small as 0.5 μm in size. Water vapor and odors are also removed, and carbon monoxide is converted to carbon dioxide. Such systems incorporate filter cartridges that are replaced periodically and are currently coming into common use.

C. Incentive Spirometry and Hand-Held Nebulizers

1. After each use, the mouthpiece and tubing connected to the mouthpiece should be rinsed with tap water and dried with a paper towel. The mouthpiece should be wrapped in a second paper towel. The towel is then secured with a twist tie.

2. In the case of an IPPB device, the manifold and nebulizer must be rinsed with tap water and dried with a paper towel. Special care must be taken to dry the nebulizer and cup.

3. Single-patient-use incentive spirometry devices must be discarded when discontinued.

4. Since in some cases IPPB devices must be used by more than one patient, precautions to guard against cross-infection are necessary.

a. When IPPB devices are used to treat more than one patient, each patient must be provided with a complete tubing manifold setup. A mainstream bacterial filter must be attached to each tubing manifold setup. After each treatment, the mouthpiece, tubing, and manifold are rinsed and dried, and the setup is reassembled and placed in a fresh paper bag marked with the patient's name and room number.

b. Patients should be carefully instructed not to exhale through permanent incentive spirometry devices. Mouthpieces must not be used by more than one patient and should be of the inexpensive type, to be disposed of when therapy is discontinued.

SUGGESTED READING

Alvarado, C. J., S. M. Stolz, and D. G. Maki. "Nosocomial P. aeruginosa Infections from Contaminated Endoscopes." Paper presented at the ASM International Symposium on Chemical Germicides, Atlanta, Ga., 27–29 July 1990 (abstr. 39). Madison: University of Wisconsin Press, 1990.

Association for the Advancement of Medical Instrumentation. *Standards and Recommended Practices.* Vol 2: *Sterilization.* Arlington: Association for the Advancement of Medical Instrumentation, 1990.

Cahill, C. K., and J. Heath. "Sterile Water Used for Humidification in Low-Flow Oxygen Therapy: Is It Necessary?" *American Journal of Infection Control* 18 (1990): 13.

Centers for Disease Control. "Nosocomial Infection and Pseudoinfection from Contaminated Endoscopes and Bronchoscopes—Wisconsin and Missouri." *Morbidity and Mortality Weekly Report* 40 (1991): 675.

Craven, D. E., et al. "Contamination of Mechanical Ventilators with Tubing Changes Every 24 or 48 Hours." *New England Journal of Medicine* 306 (1982): 1505.

Favero, M. S., and W. W. Bond. "Chemical Disinfection of Medical and Surgical Materials." In *Disinfection, Sterilization, and Preservation,* 4th ed. Edited by S. S. Block. Philadelphia: Lea and Febiger, 1991.

LaForce, F. M. "Lower Respiratory Tract Infections." In *Hospital Infections,* 3d ed. Edited by J. V. Bennett and P. S. Brachman. Boston: Little, Brown, 1992.

Occupational Safety and Health Administration. "Gluteraldehyde." *Federal Register* 54 (1989): 2464.

Rahame, F. S. "The Inanimate Environment." In *Hospital Infections,* 3d ed. Edited by J. V. Bennett and P. S. Brachman. Boston: Little, Brown, 1992.

Rutala, W. A. "APIC Guidelines for Infection Control Practice: APIC Guidelines for Selection and Use of Disinfectants." *American Journal of Infection Control* 18 (1990): 99–117.

Rutala, W. A., et al. "Disinfection Practices for Endoscopes and Other Semicritical Items." *Infection Control and Hospital Epidemiology* 12 (1991): 282.

Vallandigham, J. C., and W. G. Johanson, Jr. "Infections Associated with Endotracheal Intubation and Tracheostomy." In *Infections Associated with Indwelling Medical Devices.* Edited by A. L. Bisno and F. A. Waldvogel. Washington, D.C.: American Society for Microbiology, 1989.

Chapter 8

Maintaining a Surveillance System

CHAPTER OBJECTIVES

Upon completion of this chapter, the reader will be able to

1. describe the elements of a hospital surveillance system
2. describe the use of streak plates
3. explain the swab technique for sampling equipment
4. list the general categories of bacteria identified through the use of Gram's stain

Maintaining an effective infection control system in large part is the responsibility of the department head because that person oversees the decontamination system for the department on a day-to-day basis. Departmental infection-control systems must function as a part of the overall infection-control system developed by the infection-control committee and administered by the infection-control team or nurse.

I. The Hospital's Surveillance System

A. This system is developed by the infection-control committee and is put into effect by the infection-control team or nurse. It includes monitoring of culture reports, review of patients' charts on rounds by infection-control personnel, contacting of nurses and physicians, and review of the charts of discharged patients. Routine microbiological sampling of the environment, inanimate articles, and personnel is not considered to be effective. The exception is that all steam and ethylene oxide

(ETO) gas sterilizers should be checked at least once a week with a biological indicator.

1. In the event of a major change in a department's disinfection or sterilization procedures, for example, the purchase of new equipment such as a pasteurizer, or if an evaluation of a department's current procedure is deemed necessary by the infection-control team or nurse, the following procedures are appropriate:

   a. Sample the items after processing to evaluate the effectiveness of the decontamination procedures.

   b. Sample items randomly taken from storage to evaluate packaging and storage procedures.

   c. Return reports of laboratory analysis of samples to the department head and, if unsatisfactory, develop new procedures.

2. Nosocomial infections investigation takes place when there is an outbreak of nosocomial infections in the hospital. Intensive efforts are made by the infection-control team or nurse to discover the source of the outbreak.

   a. Patient charts are scrutinized to determine if the patients are receiving similar modes of treatment or have undergone similar diagnostic procedures. Their diagnoses, drugs that have been administered, and other factors are compared and analyzed.

   b. Selective sampling of the patient's environment, including objects and employees, is undertaken.

   c. The infection-control nurse consults with all employees who have had contact with the patients, and procedures are reviewed with department heads.

   d. Necessary changes in procedures are implemented.

3. The primary purpose of the bacteriologic laboratory in the hospital is the cultivation, isolation, and identification of pathologic microorganisms in the patient population and in the hospital environment. Familiarity with some of the methods and substances used in the laboratory is essential for the respiratory-therapy department head and supervisors.

4. Culture media are of two physical forms. If a medium is in the liquid state, it is called a broth; if it is in the solid form, agar has been added to the broth. Broths are developed differently to match the nutritional and physical needs of

various microorganisms. Agar is a carbohydrate derived from seaweed and does not serve as a nutrient for the microorganisms.

   a. Synthetic or defined media are those of which the composition is known.

   b. Nonsynthetic media, also called complex media, are those of which the exact composition is not known, and they are usually composed of tissue extracts or infusions. Nutrient broth is an example of nonsynthetic media.

   c. Media are also differentiated according to their use.

     (1) All-purpose media support the growth of most microorganisms. Most frequently, trypticase soy broth is used.

     (2) Enriched media contain nutritive supplements. The most common enriched medium is blood agar containing beef heart muscle, tryptose, salt, agar, and sheep or horse blood.

     (3) Selective media are developed with the special needs of certain microorganisms in mind and vary greatly in their composition.

     (4) Differential media are developed for the purpose of distinguishing among various genera and species of microorganisms. These, too, vary greatly in their composition.

     (5) Enrichment media contain not only specific ingredients to encourage the growth of specific microorganisms but also agents that inhibit the growth of other microbes.

     (6) Transport media are placed in plates and tubes for use in the case of a delay between taking the sample and transporting it to the laboratory. The most commonly used transport medium is Stuart's medium. Special containers are necessary for use in the cultivation and isolation of oxygen-sensitive anaerobes.

     (7) Containers used in the cultivation of obligate anaerobes include the Glas Pak, in which water and a catalyst are added to produce hydrogen and carbon dioxide that combine to form water, thus producing an anaerobic environment; the Bio Bag, consisting of a gas-impermeable bag, an ampule containing an

indicator, and a gas ampule, which are crushed, removing any gas in the bag.

B. The isolation of a single species of microorganism is called the pure culture technique. There are several methods used to obtain a pure culture.

1. Streak plates contain a small amount of agar upon which an inoculating loop is used to streak the agar surface with the microorganisms to be identified (Figure 8–1). After the streaking and incubation period, the microbes appear as colonies on the agar (Figure 8–2). Usually a second streak plate is cultivated from the first to ensure that only one kind of microorganism has been isolated.

2. The pour plate method is used in the isolation and identification of anaerobes and microaerophiles. In this technique, the microbial sample is first diluted and then placed in a sterile petri dish. Then agar is melted and poured into the dish. After incubation, colonies are found in and on the surface of the agar. This technique is most useful in evaluating milk and food.

3. Membrane filters are very thin, porous sheets of cellulose esters and other materials. In this process, fluid is passed through the filter. The filter is then placed on an agar medium, which is then incubated.

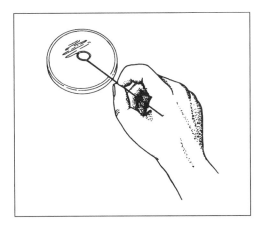

Figure 8–1 Inoculating Loop Being Used To Streak Agar in a Petri Dish.

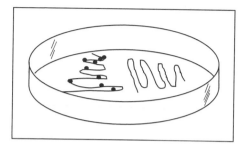

Figure 8–2 A Streak Plate. The lines indicate where the inoculating loop has been brushed against the agar. The dots indicate individual colonies of bacteria.

C. In the hospital, rapid isolation of microorganisms is essential for the speedy treatment of patients. There are several frequently used media for preliminary isolation.

1. Thioglycolate contains nutrients, a small amount of agar, and thioglycolic acid and encourages the growth of anaerobes.
2. Blood agar supports the growth of a wide range of microorganisms and also provides information about the hemolytic activities of microorganisms.
3. Eosin, methylene blue agar, and MacConkey agar inhibit the growth of gram-positive microbes and are used in the identification of gram-negative microorganisms.
4. Phenylethyl alcohol is used for the identification of gram-positive cocci.
5. Chocolate blood agar is blood agar that has been heated until it turned brown. It is often used with antibiotics.

D. Two laboratory procedures of interest to respiratory therapists because of the nature of the microorganisms that they identify are the Gram's stain and the acid-fast stain.

1. The Gram's stain is one of the most basic and important isolation procedures because it divides the bacterial world into at least four categories: gram-positive cocci, gram-negative cocci, gram-positive bacilli, and gram-negative bacilli. The Gram's stain is of no use for isolating microorganisms without cell walls. The Gram's stain procedure includes the following four steps:
   a. The primary stain is done with crystal violet, and the smear is then washed. All cells appear blue or purple.

b. The crystal violet is further fixed by the application of a mordant, which is a solution of iodine.

c. A solution of 95% alcohol is applied to decolorize the stained smear. This denatures carbohydrates, which are contained in large amounts in the walls of gram-positive organisms, and they retain the original stain. The dye is removed from the gram-negative organisms because their cell walls contain a large amount of lipids for which alcohol is a solvent.

d. Safranin is used to counterstain the smear, and the decolorized gram-negative cells take on its red color.

2. The acid-fast stain procedure is used on some bacteria, including species of *Mycobacterium* and *Nocardia* because they contain waxes and phospholipids that prevent dyes from penetrating their surfaces. Two staining techniques are used.

a. In the Kinyoun method, carbolfuchsin, a red dye, is applied for 3 minutes, then washed with water and treated with acid alcohol. A counterstain of malachite green is applied, and the specimen is again washed with water. Acid-fast organisms retain the red stain, and nonacid-fast organisms retain the green stain.

b. In the Ziehl-Neelsen test, the specimen is stained with carbolfuchsin and then heated in a flame, rinsed in acid alcohol, and methylene blue is added. Acid-fast organisms retain the red stain, and nonacid fast organisms retain the blue.

3. Other staining techniques used in the laboratory include the negative stain, in which the background of the specimen rather than the cell is stained, which shows the presence of capsules. Some stains detect the presence of flagella on a cell, or stains to detect spores.

II. The Department's Surveillance System

The respiratory-therapy department should aid the infection-control team or nurse by establishing its own sampling system in cooperation with the nurse and the laboratory, to be used when deemed necessary.

A. Sampling by Therapists

Respiratory therapists can be easily trained to obtain bacteriologic samples for evaluation. There are basically three types of samples that can be taken by therapists.

1. The use of swabs to sample equipment and the department's surfaces is the simplest sampling technique (Figure 8–3).
   a. Using aseptic technique, the swab is removed from its sterile container and rubbed on the surface to be evaluated.
   b. The swab is placed in its container, rubbed across the surface of a culture medium, and sealed.
   c. The sample is labeled with the date, type of equipment sampled, and the specific location of the swabbing; for example, the exact part of a humidifier or volume ventilator.

2. The use of broths as a culture medium is particularly useful in the sampling of tubing through which gas is passed in patient care. There are two methods.
   a. Using aseptic technique, effluent gas from the tubing is bubbled through the broth, which is stored in a suitable container. The container is labeled as described in 1, c.

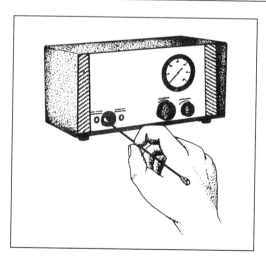

Figure 8–3 Swabbing the Exit Port of an Intermittent Positive-Pressure Breathing (IPPB) Unit for Evaluation by the Laboratory.

The broth can be either filtered through a disk for evaluation or cultured in a suitable medium.
  b. Broth can be poured into tubing, washed back and forth in the tubing, and either poured through a disk or cultured in a suitable medium. The broth must be accurately labeled as described in II, 1, c. before it is sent to the lab.
  3. The funnel-and-plate method is also simple, but sophisticated equipment is available for sophisticated testing over various amounts of time.
    a. Effluent gas is directed into a funnel leading to a plate containing culture media for 10 seconds.
    b. The funnel is removed, and the plate is covered, labeled, and sent to the laboratory.
  B. Recordkeeping
    The department head should record the results of sampling in the same general manner used by the infection-control nurse. That is, the date of the sample should be noted with the specific site and kind of object sampled, along with the status of that object. The status is
    • sampled after processing
    • sampled after pulling from storage
    • sampled in use with date that equipment was placed in use
  C. Culturing of Personnel
    Routine culturing of personnel has been shown to be time-consuming and expensive, and it produces negligible results. Culturing of employees should be done only in the case of a nosocomial infection outbreak and supervised by the infection-control team or nurse.

SUGGESTED READING

Balows, A., ed. *Manual of Clinical Microbiology.* Washington, D.C.: American Society for Microbiology, 1991.

Boyd, R. F. *Basic Medical Microbiology,* 5th ed. Boston: Little, Brown, 1995.

Brachman, P. S. "Epidemiology of Nosocomial Infections." In *Hospital Infections,* 3d ed. Edited by J. V. Bennett and P. S. Brachman. Boston: Little, Brown, 1992.

Groschel, D. H. "Air Sampling in Hospitals." *Annals of the New York Academy of Sciences* 353 (1980): 230.

Isenberg, H. D., ed. *Clinical Microbiology Procedures Handbook,* Suppl. 1. Washington, D.C.: American Society for Microbiology, 1994.

Guidelines for Prevention of Nosocomial Pneumonia

Risk Factors and Suggested Infection Control Measures for Prevention of Nosocomial Pneumonia

Risk Factors	Infection Control Measures Suggested To Prevent Nosocomial Pneumonia
Bacterial Pneumonia Host-Related: Age >65 Years Underlying illness:	
Chronic Obstructive Pulmonary Disease (COPD)	Perform incentive spirometry; positive and expiratory pressure or continuous positive airway pressure by face mask.
Immunosuppression	Avoid exposure to potential nosocomial pathogens; decrease duration of immunosuppression, such as by administration of granulocyte macrophage colony stimulating factor (GMCSF).
Depressed consciousness	Administer central nervous system depressants cautiously.
Surgery (thoracic/ abdominal)	Properly position patients; promote early ambulation; approximately control pain.
Device-Related	Properly clean, sterilize or disinfect, and handle devices; remove devices as soon as the indication for their use ceases.
Endotracheal intubation and mechanical ventilation	Gently suction secretions; place patient in semirecumbent position, i.e., 30° to 45° head-elevation; use nonalkalinizing gastric cytoprotective agent on patients at risk for stress bleeding; do not routinely change ventilator circuits more often than every 48 hours; drain and discard inspiratory-tubing condensate, or use heat-moisture exchanger if indicated.

Risk Factors	Infection Control Measures Suggested To Prevent Nosocomial Pneumonia
Nasogastric tube (NGT) placement and enteral feeding	Routinely verify appropriate tube placement; promptly remove NGT when no longer needed. Drain residual; place patient in semirecumbent position as described above.
Personnel- or Procedure-Related Cross-contamination by hands	Educate and train personnel; wash hands adequately and wear gloves appropriately; conduct surveillance for cases of pneumonia, and give feedback to personnel.
Antibiotic administration	Use antibiotics prudently, especially on high-risk intensive-care unit (ICU) patients.
Legionnaires' Disease	
Host-Related Immunosuppression	Decrease duration of immunosuppression.
Device-Related Contaminated aerosol from devices	Sterilize/disinfect aerosol-producing devices before use; use only sterile water for respiratory humidifying devices; do not use cool-mist room-air "humidifiers" without adequate sterilization or disinfection.
Environment-Related Aerosols from contaminated water supply	Hyperchlorinate or superheat hospital water system; routinely maintain water-supply system; consider use of sterile water for drinking by immunosuppressed patients.
Cooling-tower draft	Properly design, place, and maintain cooling towers.
Aspergillosis	
Host-Related Severe granulocytopenia	Decrease duration of immunosuppression, such as by administration of GMCSF; place patients with severe and prolonged granulocytopenia in protected environment.
Environment-Related Construction activity	Remove granulocytopenic patients from vicinity of construction; if not already done, place severely granulocytopenic patients in protected environment; make severely granulocytopenic patients wear a mask when they leave their protected environment.
Other environmental sources of aspergilli	Routinely maintain hospital air-handling system and rooms of immunosuppressed patients.

Risk Factors	Infection Control Measures Suggested To Prevent Nosocomial Pneumonia
Respiratory Syncytial Virus (RSV) Infection Host-Related Age <2 Years: Congenital Pulmonary/Cardiac Disease, Immunosuppression	Consider routine preadmission screening of patients at high risk for severe RSV infection, followed by cohorting of patients and nursing personnel during hospital outbreaks of RSV infection.
Personnel- or Procedure-Related Cross-contamination by hands	Educate personnel; wash hands; wear goves; wear a gown; during outbreaks, use private rooms or cohort patients and nursing personnel, and limit visitors. Place infected patients in private rooms or cohort them.
Influenza Host-Related Age >65 years: Immunosuppression	Vaccinate high-risk patients before the influenza season each year; use amantadine or rimantadine for chemoprophylaxis during an outbreak.
Personnel-Related Infected personnel	Before the influenza season each year, vaccinate personnel caring for high-risk patients; use amantadine or rimantadine for prophylaxis during an outbreak.

Source: Reprinted from Centers for Disease Control and Prevention.

Appendix B

Characteristics of the Aminoglycosides

Aminoglycoside	Principal Clinical Use	Comments
Streptomycin	Treatment of tuberculosis but always with other drugs; treatment of tularemia and plague; combined with penicillin in treatment of endocarditis caused by enterococci and viridans streptococci	Most microorganisms develop resistance to drug when used alone; therefore, it is used only under special circumstances
Kanamycin	Used primarily as a topical drug or for oral therapy	Lacks activity against pseudomonads; susceptible to inactivation by a number of aminoglycoside-modifying enzymes
Gentamicin	Widely used in treatment of infections caused by facultative and aerobic bacilli, for example, the Enterobacteriaceae	Effective against pseudomonads and most Enterobacteriaceae; resistant strains found primarily in hospitals
Tobramycin	Spectrum of activity similar to gentamicin's	More active against *Pseudomonas aeruginosa* than is gentamicin; resistant strains primarily in hospitals
Sisomicin	Spectrum of activity similar to gentamicin's	Similar to tobramycin in its activity against *P. aeruginosa*
Amikacin	Has broadest spectrum of activity of aminoglycosides; particularly effective against *Pseudomonas* species	Produced from the acylation of kanamycin; resistant to aminoglycoside-modifying enzymes; no major resistant strains detected

207

Aminoglycoside	Principal Clinical Use	Comments
Neomycin	Used primarily as a topical agent because of toxicity; activity spectrum similar to kanamycin	Occasionally administered orally as an antiseptic before bowel surgery
Fortimicin A	Activity parallels that of amikacin but has greater activity against *Serratia marcescens*	Resembles kanamycin in its poor activity against *P. aeruginosa*
Netilmicin	Resistant to enzymes that modify gentamicin and sisomicin; effective against more strains of enteric bacilli than is gentamicin	A semisynthetic derivative of sisomicin
5-Episisomicin	More active against *P. aeruginosa, S. marcescens, Providencia* species than is gentamicin	A semisynthetic derivative of sisomicin

Source: Reprinted with permission from *Basic Medical Microbiology,* R.F. Boyd, © 1995, published by Little, Brown and Company.

Characteristics of Some Important Chemotherapeutic Agents

Drug and Site of Inhibition	*Microbial Group Involved and Specific Clinical Use*
Cell wall inhibitors	
Penicillins	Bacteria; effective against gram-positive and gram-negative, depending on preparation used
Cephalosporins	Bacteria; effective against gram-positive and gram-negative, depending on preparation used
Bacitracin	Bacteria; used primarily in topical preparations because of tissue toxicity
Vancomycin	Bacteria; for staphylococcal infections that do not respond to penicillins, treatment of antibiotic-associated pseudomembranous colitis
Cytoplasmic membrane inhibitors	
Amphotericin B	Fungi; treatment of systemic fungal infections by *Candida, Histoplasma,* and *Blastomyces;* combined with flucytosine to reduce potential toxicity to kidney
Nystatin	Fungi; topical agent in treatment of *Candida* infections
Imidazoles (ketoconazole, miconazole, etc.)	Fungi; ketoconazole for systemic fungal infections but others used primarily as topical agents
Polymyxins	Bacteria; because of toxicity to kidneys, used primarily in topical preparations
Protein synthesis inhibitors	
Aminoglycosides (streptomycin, amikacin, etc.)	Bacteria
Chloramphenicol	Bacteria; toxicity reduces its use to treatment of typhoid and meningitis in which the patient is allergic to penicillins

Drug and Site of Inhibition	Microbial Group Involved and Specific Clinical Use
Erythromycin	Bacteria; absence of toxicity makes it suitable alternative to other drugs that are toxic or cause allergic reactions; drug of choice in Legionnaires' disease and pneumonia caused by *Mycoplasma pneumoniae*
Lincomycin	Bacteria; used to treat staphylococcal infections that do not respond to penicillins
Clindamycin	Bacteria and some protozoa; anaerobic pulmonary infections
Tetracyclines	Bacteria; rickettsial and chlamydial infections
Nucleic acid synthesis inhibitors	
Rifampin	Bacteria; treatment of tuberculosis, combined with other drugs
Nalidixic acid and fluoroquinolones	Bacteria; primarily in preventing gram-negative urinary tract infections in compromised patients
Flucytosine	Fungi; yeast infections (*Candida*) but also combined with amphotericin B to reduce toxicity in treatment of systemic infections
Ribavirin	Virus; respiratory syncytial virus and Lassa fever virus
Amantadine	Virus; influenza A virus infections
Idoxuridine	Virus; herpes simplex virus type 1 infections of the eye
Vidarabine	Virus; herpes zoster (shingles), herpes simplex encephalitis, and chickenpox in immunocompromised patients
Acyclovir	Virus; genital herpes infections
Zidovudine (AZT)	Virus; human immunodeficiency virus (HIV)
Antimetabolites	
Sulfonamides	Bacteria, some urinary tract infections; topical forms for burn patients; oral preparations to prevent traveler's diarrhea
Para-amino- salicyclic acid	Bacteria; only in tuberculosis
Ethambutol	Bacteria; used exclusively in treatment of tuberculosis
Trimethoprim	Bacteria; used primarily in combination with a sulfonamide, sulfamethoxazole, for treatment of hospital-associated diseases of respiratory, urinary, and gastrointestinal tracts; also used in treatment of *Pneumocystis carinii* pneumonia in AIDS patients
Isoniazid	Bacteria; tuberculosis
Nitrofurans	Bacteria, fungi, protozoa; nitrofurantoin used to prevent urinary tract infections following catheterization

Source: Reprinted with permission from *Basic Medical Microbiology*, R.F. Boyd, © 1995, published by Little, Brown and Company.

Glossary

Abscess—A localized collection of pus

Active immunity—Acquired immune status that results from an infection or immunization with vaccines

Acute—Having a short and relatively severe course

Adhesions—Components on microbial surfaces used for attachment to host cells or tissues

Aerobic—Oxygen required for growth

Agglutination—A reaction in which cells are clumped

Allergen—An antigen that elicits allergic reactions

Allergy—A hypersensitivity to animate or inanimate substances

Amphitrichous—Having one flagellum at each pole of the cell

Anabolism—Metabolic process involved in the synthesis of cell material

Anaerobic—Growing only in the absence of molecular oxygen

Anaerobiosis—Life in the absence of oxygen

Anaphylaxis—The state in which an individual is hyperactive to a given antigen

Antibiotic—A chemical compound that can inhibit or kill other microorganisms

Antibody—A glycoprotein produced by mammalian hosts in response to antigen, and which reacts specifically with that antigen

Antigen—A foreign substance capable of inducing an immunologic response

Antisepsis—The process or state that is against sepsis, that prevents the development of sepsis

Antiseptic—A chemical compound that can be used on the surface of living tissue that inhibits bacterial growth

211

Antiserum—A serum containing specific antibodies

Antitoxin—A specific antibody capable of neutralizing the exotoxin that stimulated its production

Arthropod—An invertebrate with jointed limbs

Arthrospore—An asexually produced fungal spore that is thick walled and barrel shaped

Asepsis—The avoidance of sepsis or deterrence to the development of sepsis

Aseptic—Free of living microorganisms

Atopic Allergies—Common clinical allergies in which there is a hereditary predisposition to form IgE

Atrophy—The wasting away of a tissue, organ, limb, etc.

Attenuation—Lessening; reduction of the virulence of microorganisms, as in a vaccine

Australia antigen—A viruslike antigen associated with serum hepatitis (hepatitis B); originally discovered in an Australian aborigine, hence the name

Autoclave—A sealed chamber used for steam sterilizing

Autoimmune disease—Disease in which the host system destroys its own tissue

Autolysis—Digestion of a cell by enzymes produced by that cell at the time of death

Autotroph—An organism that obtains energy by the oxidation of inorganic compounds

Auxotroph—A mutant microorganism that will grow only on minimal media supplemented with growth factors not required by the normal parent

Bacillus—An organism of the genus *Bacillus*; also used to designate rod-shaped bacteria

Bacteremia—Presence of bacteria in the bloodstream

Bactericide—An agent that kills bacteria

Bacteriocin—Antimicrobial substance produced by bacteria that kills sensitive members of related strains

Bacteriophage—A bacterial virus, sometimes referred to as phage

Bacteriostatic—An agent that inhibits the growth of bacteria

Bacteriuria—Presence of bacteria in the urine

Basidiospore—A sexually produced spore of the subdivision basidiomycotina

B cells—The lymphocyte population involved in the production of antibodies (humoral immunity)

Benign—Not malignant and subject to recovery

Biosynthesis—The building up of chemical compounds

Biotype—A strain or organism that exhibits a specific biochemical response to substrates

Blastospore—A spore formed by budding, as occurs in yeast cells

Blocking antibody—An antibody that can inhibit the activity of another antibody

Boil—A localized abscess resulting from infection of a hair follicle; also called a furuncle

Booster dose—An amount of immunogen given some time after primary immunization to sustain the immune response at a high level

Brownian movement—Dancing motion of particles in a liquid due to thermal agitation

Buboes—Lymph nodes that have become enlarged

Bulla—A blister or vesicle filled with fluid

Capneic—Requiring elevated levels of carbon dioxide for growth

Capsid—The protein coat of a virus

Capsule—A slimy envelope that surrounds certain microorganisms

Carbuncle—An infection of the skin or subcutaneous tissue containing multiple draining sinuses

Carrier—A host that harbors infectious microorganisms and can transmit them to others but shows no disease symptoms

Caseation—A type of necrosis in which the tissue resembles an amorphous mass of cheese

Catabolism—A metabolic process in which food is broken down to release energy

Catarrh—A stage during infection in which there is coughing and sneezing

Cell-mediated immunity (CMI)—An acquired immunity in which the T lymphocytes play a major role; responsible for resistance to infectious diseases, some autoimmune diseases, and certain allergies

Cellulitis—Diffuse inflammation of connective tissue

Chancre—The primary lesion of syphilis

Chemostat—An apparatus used to maintain bacterial cultures in a state of continuous division

Chemotaxis—Phenomenon of attraction of leukocytes in response to chemicals released at the site of irritation

Chemotherapeutic agents—Agents such as antibiotics and sulfa drugs, which are usually taken internally

Chemotherapy—Treatment of disease through the administration of drugs that are toxic to microorganisms

Chronic—Over a long period of time

-cidal, -cider—Suffixes meaning "to kill"

Cirrhosis—A disease of the liver

Clone—A group of identical cells or organisms derived from a single cell or organism

Coccobacillus—An oval bacterial cell resembling both coccus and rod shapes

Coccus—A spherical bacillus

Coenzyme—An organic molecule loosely bound to the enzyme and necessary for the activity of the enzyme

Colicin—A protein secreted by certain strains of *Escherichia coli* and lethal to other strains of the same species

Colitis—Inflammation of the colon

Colony—A uniform mass of cells derived from a single cell, grows on a solid surface

Commensalism—Symbiotic relationship between different species of organisms in which neither is harmed

Complement—A series of complex thermolabile plasma proteins

Condyloma—A papulelike lesion found on the vulva or anus

Conidia—Asexual fungal spores produced on specialized mycelial branches called conidiophores

Conjugation—The act of joining together; in bacteria, a process in which genetic information is transferred from one cell to another

Constitutive (enzyme)—An enzyme produced by a cell under any environmental conditions

Coproantibodies—Antibodies occurring in the intestinal tract; consist primarily of the IgA class

Coryza—Inflammation of the nasal mucosa characterized by nasal discharge and watery eyes

C-reactive protein—A plasma protein that appears in response to inflammation in the body

Culture—A population of microorganisms growing in a nutrient medium

Cytochrome—A respiratory pigment involved in oxidation-reduction reactions

Cytopathic—Characterized by pathologic change in a cell

Cytopathic effect (CPE)—Morphologic alteration of host cells that usually results in cell death

Debilitated—Characterized by loss of strength or health

Debridement—Removal of dead or damaged tissue

Definitive (final) host—The most important host; the one in which the sexually mature adult or adult stage of a parasite develops

Degermation—The removal of transient microorganisms of the skin by mechanical and chemical means

Dehydrogenation—A process in which hydrogens are removed from a compound

Dementia—Mental deterioration

Demyelination—Removal of the myelin sheath around nerve fibers

Denaturation—A process in which a macromolecule loses its configuration and often its biologic activity

Desensitization—The process of reducing one's sensitivity

Desiccate—To dry

Desquamation—Shedding of the superficial layers of skin

Detergent—A synthetic cleansing agent

Determinant group—The chemical grouping on the antigen molecule that reacts specifically with the antibody molecule

Diarrhea—Abnormal fluidity of fecal discharge

Diphtheroid—Resembling the diphtheria bacillus

Disease—An abnormal condition of the body having characteristic symptoms

Disinfectant—A substance that destroys vegetative pathogens

Dysuria—Painful urination

Ectatic—Distended

Ectopic—Not in the normal place

Eczema—An inflammatory skin disease characterized by scales and crusts as well as watery lesions

Edema—Excessive accumulation of fluid in the tissues

Empyema—Pus accumulation usually associated with the thorax

Enanthem—Eruption of a mucosal surface

Endemic—Continually present in a community

Endocarditis—Inflammation of the endocardium of the heart

Endoenzyme—An enzyme produced by a cell whose activity is associated with intracellular processes

Endogenous—Produced within the cell; coming from within

Endometritis—Inflammation of the endometrium of the uterus

Endoplasmic reticulum—A protoplasmic network of cells in higher animals and plants consisting of a continuous double-membrane system that courses throughout the cytoplasm

Endospore—A spore occurring within the cell

Endotoxin—A toxin derived from the cell wall of gram-negative bacteria

Enteric—Occurring in the gastrointestinal tract

Enterotoxin—A toxin that gives rise to gastrointestinal symptoms when ingested

Envelope—A host cell-derived membrane, containing virus-specific antigens, which is acquired during virus maturation

Epidemic—An outbreak of a disease affecting a large number of individuals in a community

Epidemiology—Science that deals with the incidence, transmission, and prevention of disease

Epizootic—An outbreak of disease affecting a large number of animals

Erythematous—Having red eruptions on the skin

Eschar—A dry mass of necrotic (dead) tissue

Etiology—Study of the causation of a disease

Eukaryotic—A cell type in which the nuclear material is bounded by a membrane

Exanthem—Eruptive disease or fever characterized by nodular eruptions on mucous membrane

Exfoliation—Shedding of layers of the skin

Exoenzyme—An enzyme secreted by the cell and associated in activity with the extracellular process

Exotoxin—Toxin produced in the cell and released into the environment

Exudate—Material (fluids, cells, etc.) that has escaped from blood vessels

Facultative anaerobes—Organisms that grow best under aerobic conditions but can grow anaerobically

Febrile—Pertaining to fever

Fermentation—An anaerobic metabolic process that utilizes an organic compound as the final electron acceptor

F factor—An episomal fertility factor that determines the sex of a bacterium

Fibrosis—Formation of fibrous tissue

Filamentous—Composed of long, threadlike structures

Fimbria—Fringe; in microbial genetics, a small projection (pilus) on the surface of bacteria

Fission—The act of splitting, a form of asexual reproduction

Fistula—An abnormal passageway providing organisms with communication between tissues during infection

Flagella—Hairlike projections on the cell that aid in locomotion

Flora—The resident organisms in a particular area

Folliculitis—Inflammation of follicles, e.g., hair follicles

Fomite—An inanimate object that may be involved in disease transmission

Fulminating—Occurring very suddenly and with intensity

Fungicide—An agent capable of destroying fungi

Furuncle—A boil

Gamete—A sex cell

Gamma globulin—A blood protein fraction with which antibodies are associated

Genetic engineering—Recombinant DNA technology in which genes are inserted into DNA of related and unrelated organisms

Genome—The complete set of hereditary factors

Genotype—The genetic constitution of an organism

Genus—A taxonomy category

Germicide—An agent that destroys pathogenic microorganisms

Germination—The sprouting of a spore and the formation of a vegetative cell

Germ tube—A hyphal element arising from a germinating spore

Globulins—A class of proteins found in the blood

Glycolysis—The anaerobic process in which carbohydrates such as glucose are oxidized to pyruvic or lactic acid

Gnotobiotic animals—Animals harboring one or more known microorganisms

Granuloma—A tumorlike mass of granulation tissue containing actively growing fibroblasts; due to chronic inflammation

Halophilic—In bacteria, requiring high concentrations of salt to maintain the integrity of the cell

Helminth—A worm

Hemagglutination—Clumping of red blood cells

Hematogenous—Derived from the bloodstream

Hematuria—Presence of blood in the urine

Hemolysin—Any agent that can cause the lysis of red blood cells

Heterotroph—An organism requiring organic material for energy and biosynthesis

Histamine—A physiologically active substance released by certain cell types, especially mast cells, affecting capillary permeability and smooth muscle contraction

Histone—A protein containing many basic amino acids and associated with the DNA of eukaryotic cells

Hydrolase—An enzyme that catalyzes the hydrolysis of compounds

Hydrolyze—To split a compound by the addition of water

Hydrops—Edema

Hyperchromic—Highly stained

Hyperplasia—Increase in the number of cells in a tissue

Hypertonic—A solution in which the concentration of solutes, e.g. NaCl, is higher outside the cell than inside the cell

Hypha (pl. hyphae)—One of the filaments that make up a fungal mycelium

Hyposensitization—A process in which an allergen is injected to reduce the allergic state

Hypotonic—A solution having a lower salt concentration than an isotonic solution

Icterus (jaundice)—A condition characterized by excess of bile pigments in the blood and tissues that leads to a yellow color of the surface integuments

Id—An allergic reaction to fungi or fungal products

Immune globulin—A preparation of purified antibody used to confer immunity

Immunity—A state of being protected, especially from microorganisms or their products

Immunogen—An antigen or a substance that induces an immunity

Immunoglobulins—A class of blood proteins with which antibodies are associated

Immunosuppressive—Inhibiting the normal immunologic response of an organism

Impetigo—A streptococcal infection of the skin

Inclusion bodies—In virus infection, the highly stainable components, usually virus, found in the cytoplasm or nucleus of the infected cell

Indigenous—Native to a particular place

Inducer—A molecule capable of stimulating the formation of compounds such as enzymes involved in cellular metabolism

Induration—A hardened area or lesion

Infection—The state or condition in which the body or part of it is invaded by a pathogenic agent that, under favorable conditions, multiplies and produces effects that are injurious. The following terms explain the various types of infection.

    Bacteremia—A transitory infection in which bacteria present in the blood are usually cleared from the vascular system with no harmful effects

    Focal—A localized site of infection from which bacteria and their products are spread to other parts of the body

    Inapparent or subclinical—An infection that does not give rise to any detectable overt manifestations

Latent—An infection that becomes apparent when the body's resistance is lowered

Local—An infection that is restricted to a confined area

Mixed—An infection caused by two or more microorganisms

Primary—An infection caused by one microbial species

Pyemia—The presence of pyogenic (pus-forming, such as staphylococci and streptococci) bacteria in the blood as they are being spread from one site to another in the body

Secondary—A primary infection complicated with a second pathogen (e.g., pneumonia following primary influenza infection)

Septicemia—A condition in which the blood serves as a site of bacterial multiplication, as well as a means of transfer of the infectious agent from one site to another

Systemic—An infection in which the microorganism can spread throughout the body, not necessarily from a localized site

Toxemia—The presence of microbial toxins in the blood

Infectious—Able to cause disease

Infectious dose (ID60, TClso)—That amount of virus required to cause a demonstrable infection in 50% of the inoculated animals or tissue culture cells, respectively

Inflammation—Nonspecific response to irritants (chemical, physical, microbial, antigens) characterized by pain, heat, redness, and swelling

Infusion—A preparation in which important components of a substance have been extracted with water

Inoculum—A substance (microorganisms, serum, etc.) introduced into the tissues or culture media

Inspissate—To thicken by evaporation

Interferon—A class of proteins produced by vertebrate cells in response to viruses, endotoxins, and certain chemicals; associated primarily with antiviral activity

Intermediate host—A host that is required in the life cycle of some parasites during which the asexual or larval stage develops

Intoxication—The state of being poisoned by a chemical, e.g., a toxin

Intradermal—Within the skin

Intubation—Insertion of a tube

In utero—Within the uterus

Invasive—Able to invade or penetrate the body

In vitro—Outside of the body; performed in artificial environments

In vivo—Within the body or within a living organism

Iodophors—Disinfectants consisting of iodine combined with a carrier molecule

Ischemia—Blood deficiency in a body part

Isoagglutinins—Antibodies specific for antigenic sites on red blood cells of the same species and causing their agglutination; also called alloagglutinins

Jaundice—See icterus

Kaposi's sarcoma—A form of skin cancer that develops a fatal form in AIDS patients

Karyotype—Chromosomal makeup of a cell

Keratitis—Inflammation of the cornea

Kernicterus—A condition associated with high levels of bilirubin in the blood that affects the nervous system

Koplik's spots—Small bluish spots surrounded by a reddened area in the mucous membrane of the mouth and characteristic of measles

Kupffer's cells—Macrophages lining the hepatic sinusoids

Labile—Unstable or susceptible to various chemical or physical agents

Latency—A state of inactivity

LD50—Lethal dose 50; refers to the dose lethal to 50% of the subjects

Leukemia—A blood disease characterized by high levels of leukocytes

Leukocidin—A substance produced by some pathogenic bacteria and toxic to white blood cells

Leukocyte—White blood cell

Leukopenia—A smaller than normal number of circulating leukocytes

L-forms—Bacteria with deficient cell walls

Lophotrichous—Having a tuft of flagella at one end of the cell

Lymphadenopathy—Infection of a lymph node

Lymphocyte—A white blood cell devoid of cytoplasmic granules, associated with immune response and chronic inflammation

Lymphoma—Any neoplasia (abnormal growth) associated with the lymph system

Lyophilization—Process of freeze-drying

Lysin—An agent (bacterial, chemical, antibody) capable of causing the destruction of cells

Lysis—Dissolution (as in cell destruction)

Lysosome—A cell organelle containing hydrolytic enzymes collectively termed acid hydrolases

Lysozyme—An enzyme that degrades murein, a component of the cell wall

Macrophage—A large mononuclear cell derived from the reticuloendothelial system and having phagocytic activity

Macula—A spot; often associated with a type of rash (macular) in which the lesion is not elevated

Malaise—A general feeling of not being well

Mast cell—A cell that is a source of vasoactive and muscle-contracting compounds, e.g., histamine, and is involved in anaphylactic reactions

Medium—A substance that provides nutrients for the growth of microorganisms

Membrane filters—Very thin filters made of cellulose esters and other materials

Meninges—Membranes that cover the brain and spinal cord

Meningitis—An inflammation of the membranes that cover the brain and spinal cord

Mesophile—A microorganism that grows best at temperatures between 20°C and 45°C

Mesosome—Involuted membrane of the bacterial cell

Metabolism—The sum total of all the physical and chemical changes that take place in a cell and maintain the cell's integrity

Metabolite—A product of metabolic processes

Microaerophile—An organism requiring less than 1 atmosphere of oxygen

Migration inhibiting factor (MIF)—A Lymphokine that prevents macrophages from leaving the site of a cell-mediated immunologic (CMI) reaction

Miliary—Resembling millet seeds; used to describe lesions

Mold—Another name for fungi that exhibit branching

Monocyte—A macrophage of the circulating blood

Monomer—The simplest molecule of a compound

Monotrichous—Having one flagellum

Morbidity—Sickness; the ratio of sick to well individuals in a community

Mordant—A chemical that when added to a dye makes it stain more intensely

Morphologic—Related to shape or structure

Mortality—Fatality; the ratio of the number of deaths to a given population in a defined situation

Mucolytic—Capable of dissolving mucus

Mucous—Secreting mucus

Mucus—Viscous liquid

Mutation—A process in which a gene undergoes structural changes

Myalgia—Pain in muscles

Mycelium—A mat of intertwining hyphae of fungi

Myocarditis—A condition involving the heart muscle (myocardium)
Necrosis—Death of tissue or cells
Nematode—Roundworm
Neonatal—Pertaining to the first 4 weeks after birth
Neoplasia—The formation of tumors
Nephrotoxic—Toxic to the kidney
Neurotoxin—Toxin that affects the nervous system
Nosocomial—Pertaining to the hospital
Nucleocapsid—A unit of viral structure consisting of a protein coat (capsid) enclosing the nucleic acid
Nucleoid—An area of DNA concentration in a bacterial cell
Obligate—Necessary or required
Oliguria—Secretion of a diminished amount of urine
Oncogenic—Having the ability to cause tumors
Ophthalmia—Inflammation of the eye
Opportunistic pathogen—A microorganism capable of infection only under the most favorable conditions
Opsonin—An antibody that prepares cells for phagocytosis
Orchitis—Inflammation of the testes
Ornithosis—An avian disease, transmissible to humans
Osmosis—Passage of fluids through a semipermeable membrane
Osteitis—Inflammation of a bone
Otitis media—Inflammation of the middle ear
Oxidation—Loss of electrons by a compound
Oxidative phosphorylation—Enzymatic addition of phosphate to Adenosine Diphosphate (ADP) to form Adenosine Triphosphate (ATP), which is coupled to the electron transport system
Ozena—Chronic inflammation of the nose
Pandemic—A worldwide epidemic
Papule—A small, firm, circumscribed raised lesion of the skin
Parasite—An organism that survives on or at the expense of another living host
Parenteral—Outside the intestine
Pasteurization—A process in which fluids are heated at temperatures below boiling to kill pathogenic microorganisms in the vegetative state
Pathogen—An organism capable of producing disease
Pathognomonic—A disease condition that is so characteristic that a diagnosis can be made from it
Peptide bond—A bond that unites two amino acids
Peptidoglycan—The relatively rigid component of most bacterial cell walls

Percutaneous—Performed through the skin
Periostitis—Inflammation of the periosteum, the specialized connective tissue covering all bones
Peritrichous—Having flagella that cover the entire bacterial surface
Permease—An enzyme found in cell membranes that transports compounds into the cell cytoplasm
Phagocytosis—The process of ingestion of foreign particles
Phagosome—A cell vacuole resulting from phagocytosis of particulate materials
Phenotype—The genetic makeup of an organism; an organism's observable properties
Phlebitis—Inflammation of a vein
Photophobia—Painful sensitivity to light
Photosynthetic—Able to convert light to chemical energy
Phototroph—An organism that utilizes light for energy
Pilus—A small protein projection on the bacterial cell involved in conjugation or adherence
Pinocytosis—The engulfment of liquid droplets by a cell
Plasma—The fluid portion of the blood containing elements necessary for clot formation
Plasma cell—Cell type regarded as the principal producer of antibodies
Plasmolysis—Shrinkage of the cell due to osmotic removal of water
Plasmoptysis—Swelling or bursting of a cell due to osmotic inflow of water
Pleomorphism—The state of having more than one form or shape
PMN—Polymorphonuclear neutrophil leukocyte
Polymerization—Formation of a polymer from monomeric molecules
Polypeptide—A polymer made up of amino acids linked by peptide bonds
Porions—Channels into cell walls for solute transport
Predisposing—Conferring a tendency
Prodromal—The early stage of a disease before symptoms appear
Prokaryotic—Characterized by lack of nuclear membrane and organelles (e.g., bacteria and blue-green algae)
Properdin—A bactericidal protein component of the blood
Prophylaxis—Protection, e.g., against disease
Proteolytic—Able to break down proteins
Protoplast—A viable bacterial cell without its cell wall
Prototroph—An organism capable of synthesizing cell material from inorganic compounds
Provirus—Virus integrated into host chromosomes and transmitted from one generation to another

Pruritus—Itching

Psittacosis—An avian disease, transmissible to humans

Psychrophile—A microorganism that grows best at temperatures between 0°C and 20°C

Puerperal—Related to the period after childbirth

Purpura—Hemorrhage in the skin or mucous membrane

Purulent—Associated with the formation of pus

Pus—A thick yellow fluid that is produced by inflammation consisting primarily of leukocytes and serum

Pustule—An elevated lesion filled with pus

Putrefaction—Decomposition of proteins resulting in foul odors

Pyocin—Bacteriocin produced by *Pseudomonas aeruginosa*

Pyogenic—Pus forming

Pyrogen—An agent that induces fever

Quarantine—To detail or isolate individuals because of suspicion of infection

Quellung reaction—A test in which the bacterial capsule swells as a result of combining with a specific antibody

Reagin—The nonprotective antibody found in the blood and produced in response to a number of different diseases; also, the antibody of immunoglobulin class IgE, involved in anaphylaxis and atopic allergies

Recombination—A process in genetics in which information is exchanged

Recrudescence—Recurrence of symptoms after their abatement

Replication—A duplication process requiring a template

Repressible (enzyme)—An enzyme whose synthesis can be decreased by certain metabolites

Reticuloendothelial system (RES)—A network of phagocytic cells produced and residing in the bone marrow, spleen, lymph nodes, and liver of vertebrates

Rheumatoid factor—A distinctive gamma globulin found in the serum of patients with rheumatoid arthritis

Rhinitis—Inflammation of the nose

Rhizoid—A filamentous appendage by which organisms such as fungi attach themselves to the soil

Ribosome—A ribonucleoprotein particle found in the cell cytoplasm and involved in protein synthesis

Ringworm—A common name for ring-shaped patches appearing anywhere on the body surface and caused by a special group of fungi called dermatophytes

Roundworm—Worms that are round or oval in cross section

Rubella—German measles

Rubeola—Measles

Sanitization—A process that reduces the number of microorganisms on inanimate objects and in the environment to a safe level as judged by public health standards

Saprophyte—An organism that derives its nourishment from dead or decaying material

Sarcoma—A solid tumor growing from derivatives of embryonal mesoderm such as connective tissue, bone, muscle, and fat

Scrofula—A tuberculosis of the lymph glands

Secretory IgA—A class of immunoglobulins that appear in secretions of epithelial surfaces such as saliva

Sepsis—A toxic condition resulting from the presence of microbes or microbial products in the body

Septicemia—A systemic disease in which microorganisms multiply in the bloodstream

Septum—A dividing wall or partition

Sequela—A morbid (abnormal) condition that develops as a consequence of a disease

Serology—The study of antigen-antibody reactions in vitro

Serotype—A taxonomy subdivision of microorganisms based on the kind of antigens present

Serum—The clear portion of the blood minus the factors necessary for clotting

Slow virus—A virus that causes subacute or chronic disease having a long incubation period that lasts several weeks to years before the onset of clinical symptoms

Smear—A film of material such as a bacterial suspension spread on a glass slide

Snuffles—The nasal discharge from mucous patches associated with syphilis

Spectrophotometer—An instrument used to measure the absorption of light in test liquids

Spheroplast—A cell wall-deficient bacterium that retains part of the wall material

Spikes—Surface projections of varying lengths spaced at regular intervals on the virus envelope

Spirochete—A corkscrew-shaped bacterium

Splenomegaly—Enlargement of the spleen

Spondylitis—Inflammation of the vertebra

Sporangiospores—Asexual fungal spores produced in a sac called a sporangium

Spore—The resistant form of a bacterium derived from the vegetative cell; the reproductive cell of certain organisms

Sporicide—An agent that destroys spores

Sporogenesis—Production of spores

-static, -stasis—Suffixes denoting inhibition or inactivation

Stem cell—A precursors cell that can develop into functionally and morphologically different cell types

Sterilization—The process that destroys all living microorganisms

Stomatitis—Inflammation of oral mucosa

Street virus—The virulent type of rabies isolated in nature from domestic or wild animals

Streptolysin—A hemolysin produced by streptococci

Subacute—Between acute (short course) and chronic (persisting over a long period)

Subclinical—Without clinical manifestations of the disease

Substrate—A specific compound acted on by an enzyme

Superinfection—A new infection caused by an organism different from that which caused the initial infection

Suppurative—Pus forming

Surfactant—An agent that reduces surface tension

Syndrome—A group of symptoms that characterize a disease

Synergism—A phenomenon in which the action of two components together is more than that of either one alone

Synthesize—To build up a chemical compound from its individual parts

Systemic—Relating to the entire organism and not any individual organ

T cells—Thymus-dependent lymphocytes involved in cell-mediated immunity

Taxonomy—The classification into distinct categories based on some suitable relationship between groups or individual organisms

Temperate phage—A nonvirulent bacteriophage

Template—A mold for the synthesis of new material

Teratogenic—Able to induce abnormal development and congenital malformation

Thermolabile—Sensitive to heat

Thermophiles—Microorganisms growing best at temperatures between 45°C and 70°C

Thrombosis—Formation of a clot in a blood vessel

Thrombocytopenia—Decrease in the number of blood platelets
Thrush—A fungal infection involving the oral mucous membrane
Tincture—An alcoholic solution of a particular substance, e.g., tincture of iodine
Tinea—A name applied to fungal infections of the skin
Titer—The concentration of animate or inanimate agents in a medium
Tolerance—The lack of response to a specific antigen allowing the antigen to persist
Toxemia—A condition in which toxins are in the blood
Toxin—A usually organic substance produced by living organisms that is poisonous
Toxoid—A modified exotoxin that has been treated to destroy its toxicity
Transcription—The formation of messenger RNA from a DNA template
Transduction—The transfer of bacterial genetic information from one cell to another by a virus
Transferase—An enzyme that catalyzes the exchange of functional groups between compounds
Trismus—Spasm of the masticatory muscles resulting in difficulty in opening the mouth (lockjaw)
Trophozoite—The active vegetative stage of a protozoon
Tropism—The involuntary movement of an organism toward or away from a stimulus
TSS—Toxic shock syndrome, caused by *S. aureus*
Tubercle—A nodule
Tuberculoprotein (tuberculin)—Protein extract derived from Mycobacterium tuberculosis
Tumor—A new growth of tissue in which the multiplication of cells is uncontrolled; a swelling
Ulcer—A circumscribed area of inflammation characterized by necrosis and found in the epithelial lining of a surface
Urticaria—A vascular reaction of the skin characterized by elevated patches (wheals)
Vaccine—A suspension of organisms usually killed or attenuated and used for immunization
Varicella—Chickenpox
Variola—Smallpox
Vascular—Containing blood vessels
Vector—A carrier of pathogenic microorganisms
Vegetative—Concerned with the growing stage of a microorganism as opposed to the spore state

Venereal—Transmitted by sexual contact

Vesicle—A blister

Viremia—Presence of virus in the bloodstream

Virion—A complete virus particle consisting of a core of nucleic acid and a protein capsid

Viroid—An infectious subviral particle consisting of nucleic acid without a protein capsid

Virulence—The relative ability of an organism to cause disease

Wheal—A flat elevated area of skin caused by edema of underlying tissue

Yeast—A unicellular fungus

Zoonosis—A disease of animals that can be transmitted to humans

Index

H

Halogens, 145–146
Hand washing
  exceptions for, 162
  importance of, 20, 153
  indications for, 161
  lotion for, 162
  in nursery, 163
  routine, 161–162
  technique, 160–161
Hansen's disease, 71–72
HDCV (human diploid cell virus), 99
Health care costs, impact of nosocomial
  infections on, 7
Heat sensitivity, 138
Heating devices, 187–188
Helicobacter pylori, 77
Hemolytic-uremic syndrome, 57
Hemophilus ducreyi, 65
Hemophilus influenzae
  drug-resistant strains, 65
  nonencapsulated, 65
  type B (HIB), 64–65
Hemorrhagic fever viruses, 99–101
Hemorrhagic fever with renal syndrome
  (HFRS), 101
HEPA filters, 19, 143
Hepatitis viruses
  A, 106–108
  B, 107, 108–110
  C, 107, 110
  D, 107, 110
  E, 107, 110
Herd immunity, 5
Herpangina, 95
Herpes labialis, 88
Herpes simplex virus (HSV)
  type 1 infections, 87, 88
  type 2 infections, 87, 88–89
Herpesviruses, 86–90
Herpetic encephalitis, 88
Herpetic whitlows, 89
Hexachlorophene, 145
HFRS (hemorrhagic fever with renal
  syndrome), 101
HHV-6 (human herpesvirus-6),
  89–90

High-efficiency particulate air filters
  (HEPA filters), 19, 143
Histoplasmodium capsulatum, 115
Histoplasmosis, 115
HIV (human immunodeficiency virus),
  68, 103–106
Hookworms, 131
Horizontal transmission, 5, 84, 105
Hospital. *See also* Hospital personnel
  critical-care areas in, 18–19
  department heads, 24
  employee health service, 22–24
  employee health service of, 22–24
  epidemiology, 9–10
  infections acquired in. *See* Nosocomial
    infections
  physical facilities, 16–19, 22
  as special environment, 16–21
  supplies. *See* Equipment/supplies
  surveillance system, 195–200
Hospital personnel
  communicable disease evaluation in,
    23
  culturing of, 202
  hand washing for. *See* Hand washing
  as nosocomial infection source, 20
  staph lesions, 43
Host factors, 2, 12
HRIG (human rabies immune globulin),
  99
HSV (herpes simplex virus), 87–89
HTLV (human T lymphotropic viruses),
  104
Human diploid cell virus (HDCV), 99
Human herpesvirus-6 (HHV-6), 89–90
Human immunodeficiency virus (HIV),
  68, 103–106. *See also* AIDS
Human papillomaviruses (HPV), 90–91
Human rabies immune globulin (HRIG),
  99
Human T lymphotropic viruses (HTLV),
  104
Humans, relationship with microorgan-
  isms, 28–29
Humidifiers, 185–186
Hydrogen ion concentration, microbial
  growth and, 38
Hydrophobia, 98